43 days.

a legacy of survival, strength & resilience

by tansy lederhaus

Disclaimers: To the best of my ability, this book is a factual account of my personal experiences regarding the timeframe of the course of events. Because of my condition during that time, I have no memory of the days leading up to the crash, the crash itself, or nearly two weeks afterward. To help put the pieces together, portions of this story are reconstructed from the recollection of others, medical records and my own later understanding of what occurred. While every effort has been made to portray these events accurately and respectfully, some details may reflect perceptions and interpretations of those involved. Names and identifying characteristics may have been changed to protect the privacy of individuals, but the heart of the story remains exactly as it happened.

Paperback ISBN 979-8-9947466-0-8
Hardcover ISBN 979-8-9947466-1-5
LCCN 2026905531

Published in the United States of America
By The Cheeky Scribe in Calumet Michigan, USA

Photography: Tim Sweet & Tansy Lederhaus
Cover Design: Tansy Lederhaus
Chapter Art: Dreamstime.com
Internal Book Formatting: The Cheeky Scribe

www.shop43days.com

Printed in the USA
Illustrated Edition

For my two best friends, both gone too soon.

To Sarah-
You were taken in an instant, but your memory has never left.

To my mom, Julie-
You carried me through the nightmare. You were my anchor, my advocate, my everything when I couldn't fight for myself.

This book is for both of you; because without you, there wouldn't be a story to tell.

acknowledgements

I want to thank my dad for keeping a detailed journal of every aspect of the crash, hospitalization and my recovery. Without this, I would know so little. I did choose to eliminate several entries from his journal that did not make it to my book. Some things are just meant for family and not for the rest of the world.

I want to thank everyone who graciously responded to my many reach outs to have your names included in my story. I wanted it to remain as authentic as possible.

Thank you to those of you who shared their memories with me during the time I didn't have memories of my own.

Thank you to those who agreed to put your thoughts and feelings on paper to be included in this book.

Thank you to my friends and family who read through several drafts, assisted with editing and gave their recommendations.

"Out of suffering have emerged the strongest souls; the most massive characters are seared with scars."

~ Kahlil Gibran

contents

preface

Nobody expects their life to end on a typical day.

I wasn't doing anything unsafe or perilous. I wasn't risk-taking or defying the odds. I was simply driving. I was just trying to get from one place to another, like any other day.

And then everything changed.

The crash was devastating. I don't remember the collision. I don't remember the sirens or the sounds of crumpled metal. But I do know this; I nearly died that day. I was given less than one percent chance of survival.

I lived.

But Sarah didn't.

That statement still takes my breath away. Sarah, who had her whole life ahead of her with limitless potential... Sarah, who sat alongside me in the car... her life ended. Mine, somehow, didn't. That reality is ruthless. It's harsh. It's complex. It's the anguish beneath the scars.

This book isn't just about a car crash. It's about the forty-three days that followed; the days I spent in a hospital bed barely clinging to life. The days I spent in the operating room with surgeons. The days where I was kept alive by machines and more than one hundred units of donated blood. It's about the pain, the grief, the prayers and the dedication. It's about survival ...when survival felt irretrievable.

It's about what it means to live. To live when someone else doesn't get the chance. It's about living with purpose.

I wrote this book because I needed to. I wrote it to remember, to honor and to process the trauma that doesn't show up in X-rays. I wrote it for Sarah. I wrote it for the ones who loved her. I wrote it for anyone who's lost or hurting. Anyone who's ever been given a second chance and doesn't quite know what to do with it. Anyone who needs another opportunity or a new beginning.

I wrote this book for the families sitting in hospital waiting rooms and for the doctors, nurses, paramedics and blood donors who save lives every day.

This is my story. It's raw. It's authentic. And it begins on the day my life almost slipped away, with the long, harrowing, remarkable journey that followed.

Welcome to 43 days.

introduction

I grew up in Clintonville, a small town in east central Wisconsin. At the time, I lived with my parents, Tim and Julie Sweet, who were married after being friends and began dating toward the end of college.

My mom was a registered nurse who had experience in several areas of nursing including hospital, clinic and long-term care administration. My dad was a third-grade teacher at the local school district; he was my third-grade teacher too.

I have a brother named Camden who is three years younger than I; we call him Cam.

My parents were both nature lovers and instilled that appreciation in my brother and me. We lived next to the Clintonville golf course in a log home that my parents built. We had a lot of privacy and enjoyed the nature that was all around us.

At the time of the crash, I had been dating a young man named Brian for the past several years.

At some point, I acquired the nickname, Tawny. I'm pretty sure it came from someone mispronouncing my unusual name when I was born, and it's kind of stuck. My name "Tansy," and nickname "Tawny," are used interchangeably in this story.

A tansy is a fragrant plant from the daisy family with yellow, button-like flowers and feathery leaves. It grows locally, even in my yard. Some, like me, refer to it as a wildflower, while others refer to it as an herb, a weed or even invasive. The given name Tansy is a nature name, taken directly from the flower, with meanings that include immortality, tenacity and resilience, which symbolize a person's inner strength and ability to endure challenges.

Sarah and I became fast friends when we met in elementary school. We had been nearly inseparable ever since. Sarah was the kindest, friendliest person I knew. She loved spending time with her friends, playing softball and participating in choir. She sang every day, either in her room with the music blaring, in the car or while walking down the hall to class. We were big fans of pop music from the 90's, including every boy band. The first concert we went to together was Hanson.

She was a great writer, enjoyed taking photos and loved learning about the ocean. We spent many late nights on the trampoline talking, perfecting our flips and performing dance routines. We enjoyed doing photoshoots together and making movies and dance videos. We had our futures all mapped out and planned to go to college together.

We had just finished our junior year and had elaborate plans for the summer going into our senior year of high school.

And it all changed the afternoon of June 12, 2002. Sarah and I had finished our six-hour shift at A&W and were planning to travel to Green Bay together to get my new car.

I typically drove. I don't know why, I just did. Maybe because I knew the way. We made it about six minutes out of town on a state highway when our lives changed forever. Shortly after 4:00 PM, we were involved in a severe car crash at the age of seventeen.

I don't remember much in the days leading up to the crash or the crash itself, but thanks to my dad, who kept a detailed journal and took photos, I'm able to piece things together.

I have written this story based on my memories of what occurred, what I've been told by medical professionals, close friends and family and my dad's journal entries. His journal entries are in *italics*, dated and timed. My memories are woven throughout.

chapter one

the crash

When people talk about car crashes, they often focus on the moment of impact. But for me, the most important moment came after, in what medical professionals call the "golden hour."

The golden hour is the first 60 minutes after severe trauma. Every decision made, every second that passes can mean the difference between life and death.

In my golden hour, I didn't have the option of knowing what was happening. I was unconscious. My body was badly broken and bleeding. But while I was alone in the dark, others were working together in the light. Paramedics and nurses made split-second, lifesaving decisions. The hospital team stood ready. And long before I ever needed it, people donated blood. Blood that would end up saving my life.

Day 1

Wednesday, June 12, 2002

4:18 PM Clintonville ambulance receives a call. The car the girls were driving in hits the back end of a semi near the intersection of a state highway and a county road.

My theory is that Tansy saw a semi in the right-hand lane and was planning to pass it. When she was beyond the point of stopping, she sees that the semi is making a left-hand turn. Tansy jams on the brakes and attempts to avoid the semi but instead smashes into it.

Sarah was killed instantly. Tansy received life threatening injuries.

Sarah and I were driving a 1991 Mercury Cougar that didn't have airbags. Both of us were wearing our seatbelts.

A Navarino First Responder was among the first people to come upon the accident. Clintonville Area Ambulance Service was advised there were two females in the car with injuries. The Embarrass First Responders were paged, as well as Clintonville Fire Department, with their Jaws of Life.

I was later told that Sarah and I were both found draped over one another, both still belted in, with my torso over hers, as if to shield her from the impact.

Jason Selwitschka, who served on both the volunteer fire department and the ambulance service for ten years at that point, shared the following with me:

June 12, 2002, is a day I will never forget. That afternoon, I responded to a motor vehicle accident that left an indelible mark on my career and my heart.

In a small town like Clintonville, you always asked yourself the same question as you approached a scene: "Who is it? Who am I about to see?" Often, you knew the patient or their family. That knowledge brought extra weight, because in those moments you weren't just treating a patient—you were caring for a neighbor, a friend, or a classmate's daughter.

I remember leaning into the car, reaching for her hand, and saying quietly, "Hey, we're here for you. We're going to help you. You're not alone." In emergency medicine, so much of what we do is technical—checking pulses, securing airways, following the ABCs—but the human connection matters just as much. Sometimes what a patient needs most in that moment is to hear that they are not facing this alone.

Very quickly, the seriousness of the crash became clear. In rural Wisconsin, an hour away from the nearest trauma center, we knew this was beyond ground transport. That meant one thing: Theda Star. We called for the helicopter, knowing that even if we weren't certain, it was always better to have them in the air.

I'll never forget the moment dispatch radioed in: "The helicopter is ten minutes out." That single update set the pace for everything that followed. It framed how quickly the extrication had to move, how we sequenced our care, how we kept the golden hour in sharp focus. In trauma care, every decision, every move, every second matters. Our job was to make sure she was packaged, stabilized, and ready for the flight crew the moment those rotors touched down.

And then, you hear it. Before you ever see it, you hear the thrum of the helicopter blades in the distance. That sound brings both relief and urgency—relief because you know advanced help is near, and urgency because you have only minutes left to finish what must be done.

We made the handoff, transferred her to the flight crew, and then stood back as she was loaded onto the helicopter. And then came the second sound, that unforgettable sound of the helicopter lifting off, carrying her away toward definitive care. That's when the emotions hit. Standing on that road, watching it rise into the sky, you pray. You pray she survives.

Debbie Struble was the EMT with Clintonville Area Ambulance who attended to me. She echoed what

Jason had said and told me that once they got the call and heard that this was a crash between a semi and a car, they called for air assistance right away.

Debbie said when they arrived at the scene, she immediately went to the driver's side of the vehicle. She noticed that the windshield was broken, "spidered" as they called it, from being struck from the inside. She said I was slumped over and making gurgling noises. She initially held my head and neck to secure my airway and cervical spine.

They cut the seat belt and used a large brace to stabilize my body as they removed me from the vehicle. She said she looked over, and one of the men standing on the passenger side shook his head, indicating that Sarah was not alive.

The other EMT at the scene, Lisa Olmsted, noticed I had gum in my mouth. They removed the gum and were able to keep my airway open. They used a bag valve mask to ventilate me.

Debbie recalls my obvious injuries: a head injury, bruising on my chest and abdomen and a compound fracture of my left leg.

Both Sarah and I were wearing our A&W uniforms: red polo shirts, khaki shorts and Van's shoes. We looked the same. We were both 17-year-old females wearing the same clothes. We were bloody and unable to communicate who was who. I was driving Sarah's car.

4:27 PM Theda Star helicopter received a call for assistance. Jon Hagen, flight nurse, told us Tansy was very incoherent at the scene. He got right up in her face; she made brief eye contact. Then her eyes focused on nothing. They started two IVs. She pulled out one of them. They intubated her.

Jon later told me I was fighting and screaming. I had broken both of my legs. Jon shared with me that I tried lifting my legs off the stretcher. He said the effort caused my legs to bend at an unnatural angle as my fractured femurs were evident.

I was flown to Theda Clark Regional Medical Center in Neenah on an eighteen-minute helicopter ride. During the flight, Jon recalls the color literally draining out of my body. He said it was a bright, sunny day and I was so pale. He didn't think they'd get me to the trauma center alive. I arrived at the level II trauma center at 5:37 PM. The trauma center just opened on June 4th.

6:30 PM A social worker at Theda Clark called our home. Julie answered and lost it. We went searching for Camden on the golf course. Julie notified her parents. They immediately went to the ER to see Tansy being wheeled into surgery. Our drive to Neenah seemed to take forever. Julie kept trying to hail Carol and

Duane on her cellphone. (Randy later tracked them down.)

I can just imagine this nightmare unfolding in my home: my mom completely losing it on the phone when she hears what happened, and my dad having to take over. I can visualize them frantically trying to find my 14-year-old brother so they could all get to Theda Clark to be with me. Both sets of grandparents lived in Neenah just minutes from the hospital.

Around this same time frame, my friends were finding out about the car crash too. Brian and several of his friends were at football practice. Two of our girlfriends showed up and informed them of what had happened. Practice was canceled and eventually many of our friends went over to Sarah's house to be with her dad.

My friend Lisa recalls getting to Sarah's dad's house and seeing Brian sitting off to the side. She said he was red-faced and had obviously been crying. She asked him if he knew whether I was alive. She said all he could say was "I don't know. I don't know."

7:45 PM Finally, we arrived at the ER. An ER physician explained Tansy's condition: two broken legs (one compound fracture), an injured spleen, and a very badly damaged liver. She lost so much blood that she almost bled to death (was bleeding clear fluid).

I was in surgery before my parents got to Theda Clark, so they didn't get to see me initially. As soon as my parents arrived, my mom questioned the emergency room staff about how they knew that the girl they had in surgery was me and not Sarah, since we were both wearing the same clothes. They showed her the clothes they cut off me at the scene. This didn't help as it was my A&W uniform, and she knew we were both dressed the same. Then they showed her my undergarments. That's when she knew it was me.

> *Surgery could last 3-4 hours to stop the bleeding. Dr. Kevin Wasco, a trauma surgeon, saw us in an hour. They were unable to control the bleeding. Her liver was in very serious condition. They removed her spleen. Her injuries could be fatal.*

Dr. Wasco and Dr. Georgen were the trauma surgeons on duty when I arrived. Dr. Georgen later explained, "She was so unstable that we had no choice but to bring her to the operating room. When we opened her abdomen, it was a tidal wave of blood. She lost a tremendous amount of blood."

My internal injuries were caused by the seat belt. I had a grade V injury to my spleen resulting in a splenectomy, which is the removal of the spleen. I had a grade V liver laceration which was the cause of the continued hemorrhaging once my spleen was removed. I had bilateral pulmonary contusions, eventually leading to pleural effusions and the need for chest tubes. I had a closed head injury from hitting the steering wheel or windshield. I had an open left midshaft comminuted femur fracture and a closed right midshaft femur fracture.

Due to the severity of my injuries, I was placed in a drug induced coma.

My bilateral femur fractures were not considered emergent compared to the rest of my injuries. Dr. Sears, my orthopedic surgeon, later told me that my femur fractures were frankly the least of many concerns. The stress of moving me to the operating room to repair them immediately, which was their usual protocol, was deemed too risky at the time. Definitive repair was completely off the table as an option. Instead, he placed traction pins initially for skeletal traction. This involved screwing pins into my distal femur, just above my knees, to which twenty-pound weights were attached, allowing for proper alignment of the fractures temporarily.

10:00 PM Bleeding couldn't be controlled. The situation continues to worsen.

Carol and Duane arrive.

Years later, when I saw copies of my medical records the lowest recorded hemoglobin was 4. On average, a normal hemoglobin level for women is between 12 and 15. Hemoglobin is the part of red blood cells that carries oxygen from the lungs to the body's tissues and organs. It's crucial for survival.

Day 2

June 13, 2002

12:00 midnight- Hospital chaplain KC Schuler and a social worker remain with us. Camden goes to sleep in a little room in the critical care unit (CCU) waiting room. Pastor Vanman appears. He says a prayer- helps me accept Christ. Very emotional and intense. Doctors are attempting a last-ditch effort to control bleeding- will try to insert a coil in the artery feeding the liver- procedure could take as long as seven hours.

Pastor Vanman's powerful prayer ends as Dr. Wasco materialized in the darkened waiting room. He can't explain it, but the bleeding stopped on its own.

I've heard this part of the story so many times, and it still gives me chills. This must've been impossible for my parents. "A last-ditch effort." I was back in the operating room with surgeons, again, in an effort to stop the bleeding. I can picture gauze after gauze turning red, soaked with my blood, faster than they could replace it.

And suddenly...the bleeding stopped.

Now, as a parent myself, I can't help but think about what my mom and dad went through in those early morning hours. The fear. The hopelessness. The uncertainty of whether their child would make it. It's almost unbearable for me to imagine, yet it's part of my story.

> *2:00 AM Tansy stabilizes. Lab results indicate normal levels. Julie and I try to catch a few winks. We continue to check on Tansy every hour.*
>
> *9:00 AM Grandma Sweet stops by to visit.*
>
> *11:00 AM Tansy remains stable. About 20 of her friends appear with Debbie and Charlotte. They stay for three hours. Julie takes many of them back to see Tansy. Randy and Elisa, Morris and Jean, Heather, Nancy and Rodney, an almost constant stream of visitors come to give their support.*
>
> *Many people are praying in Clintonville. Visitors reported many kids thought both Tansy and Sarah had died.*

My friend Lisa N. shared her memories of the first time she and several of our friends visited me in the critical care unit. She said my mom would bring one visitor back to my room at a time. Brian was the first friend to go back to see me. She remembers my mom sitting next to Brian, talking to him with her hand resting on his shoulder in a comforting way. She recalls how strong my mom was during this time.

As I was writing this book, I specifically asked Brian what he remembered from twenty-three years ago. Hearing the news about the crash, the visit to Sarah's dad's house, his first time seeing me in the hospital hooked up to machines, not looking anything like me. His recollection of the events following the crash is very limited, likely due to his mind blocking traumatic memories as a protective mechanism. His own kind of survival.

When it was Lisa's turn to go back to see me, my mom told her that I wouldn't look like myself. She recalls walking over to my bed and my mom running her fingers through my hair and encouraging her to hold my hand, which she said she did.

After a few minutes, they went back to the waiting room together. My mom looked at Lisa and asked her if she was feeling okay as she was pale and leaning against the wall. Lisa said she was dizzy and proceeded to slide down the wall and pass out. She woke up, and my mom was there with her. My mom asked her if she'd eaten or had enough to drink that day. She hadn't.

Back in the waiting room, my mom apparently discussed the importance of everyone taking care of themselves by staying fed and hydrated. They were all in this together, navigating the trauma of losing Sarah and visiting their critically injured friend in the stressful environment of the hospital.

Lisa tells me our group of friends spent hours upon hours at the hospital, mostly in the waiting room, sometimes talking and reminiscing, but frequently silent.

Our classmates put two memorial crosses at the crash site initially because it was thought that both Sarah and I had been killed. Eventually, one was removed when it was known that I had survived. Lisa said there was a lot of confusion at first about who had survived.

> *5:00 PM A friend's mom prepared supper for us. Julie wouldn't leave the hospital, so we brought her supper here.*
>
> *6:30 PM More visitors for Tansy; Angie M. and friends, Steve and Abby. Tansy remains stable.*
>
> *10:30 PM Everyone went home. Tansy is holding her own. Julie and I got some sleep.*

During these first several days, I was in a drug induced coma. While my body was lying still in a hospital bed, my mind was on its own journey. I wasn't aware of what was going on, but I knew something was not right. I had strange, vivid dreams, so real that I can still picture the colors, smells, places and feelings they carried twenty-some years later.

I dreamt that I was in a room with many beds, like a recovery room. The room specifically looked like my Grandma and Grandpa Sweet's extra bedroom; something decorated from the 70's. I had PVC pipe-like tubes coming out of me in several areas. There were various people around, but no one was specifically talking to me, and I didn't necessarily recognize anyone. I could hear a lot. I couldn't talk. I was wondering where Sarah was. I was surprisingly calm and took everything in.

Day 3

June 14, 2002

2:00 AM Blood pressure and urinary output improving.

7:30 AM Tansy is getting plasma products in preparation for her surgery.

10:50-12:30 PM Tansy goes to surgery to have packing removed from her liver. The incision is left gaping open, increasing the size of her chest and belly- giving more room for her lungs and kidneys. The good thing about the surgery was she didn't start bleeding.

6:00 PM Dialysis has started.

Earlier today a doctor did not paint a very optimistic picture. "She's minute-by-minute." Dr. Wasco said, "On Wednesday night her chances to live were about 1-100 or 1-200. She's a fighter. She's hanging on." I prefer Wasco's attitude. He's a fighter, too. I'm glad he's on our side.

Continuous renal replacement therapy (CRRT), a specialized form of dialysis for critically ill patients, was started for acute renal failure to help my kidneys filter the excess fluid from my body. I gained almost one hundred pounds of fluid weight, nearly doubling my weight at the time. I developed stretch marks from the rapid weight gain. During this time, my parents and other visitors affectionately referred to me as the Michelin Man. My face and lips look incredibly swollen in the photos.

Day 4

June 15, 2002

3:30 AM Tansy's nurse, Sherry, wakes us to warn us that her condition has worsened. Blood pressure is dropping, and things don't look good.

Julie and I read Tansy the messages in the Steno Book from her visitors.

We call Pastor Vanman to tell him of the set back. Request nurses to call in Chaplain KC to come in.

Camden is very upset.

One of my most cherished photos is from what I'd imagine was this moment. My mom is kneeling on a pillow at my bedside. She has her hand on my face. The huge CRRT machine, ventilator and at least 8 IV pumps (my life support) are in the picture. The covers are pulled up to my shoulders, but you can see how distended my abdomen is underneath the blanket. Traction is visible at the end of my bed keeping my bilateral femur fractures in alignment. The look on my mom's face is one of pure debilitation, grief and a refusal to give up on me.

Sherry was often my nurse while I was in the critical care unit. She later shared with me what an exhausting time this was when they couldn't get my blood pressure to stabilize. She told me how tired my mom was. I have a photo of the two of them, and my mom looks so defeated. The following is a memory Sherry wrote for me to include in this book.

For Tansy

God is carrying you....

A vivid memory of Tansy as I cared for her in the ICU during a critical time. It levels me, takes my breath, even today.

It had been days of Tansy having ups and downs with her medical state. I encouraged her parents to rest. I promised them, "if she's not doing well, I will find you." And then, it happened. During the earliest am hours of the night. Tansy was slipping away from us. Her blood pressure, perfusion, oxygenation; all were deteriorating after days of holding on. She was in a chemically induced coma. Numerous vasoconstrictors infusing at maximum dosages and CRRT providing volumes of fluid every hour. Her lungs and digits; fingers and toes, compromised. A situation of extremis, even by critical care standards.

I woke her parents who were in the waiting room. A tone of pure exhaustion. Her mom placed a pillow on the floor. She knelt on it at Tansy's bedside. Leaning into her to be as close as possible amongst the large equipment sustaining her life. Her dad, slid to the floor. Testimony of love, all be it during a time of duress.

For a moment, my heart broke. Then, as many health care professionals are familiar, I shifted my thoughts to focus on the tasks at hand. Monitors alarming. IV pumps humming with the speed of rapid infusion. Triple checking all elements, ensuring maximum potential, including the CRRT machine delivering liters of fluid/ hour. What else?!... The ventilator. That's it! I called Dr. Whiteside; a man I trusted with all things I held dear. I told him, "Tansy's not doing well" and requested a novel ventilator change. A risk to her delicate pulmonary status. He paused. Silence. And then said, "Ok. Do it, but you page me the second her oxygenation falls." True to his calling and dedication. The changes were made. Then... the waiting. I prayed. I wrote in the notebook as her parents requested. "God is carrying you." I felt it. A calm, peaceful feeling. God's presence, lifted with the power of prayer and the love of her family. I wanted to hold the time as long as I could to give her what she needed to turn the situation around.

And then, the monitor blips and alarms announcing her critical state, stopped. With the grace of our Lord, she did it! She turned a corner. Her blood pressure rose, her oxygenation improved. She stabilized.

My next memory is Dr. Whiteside walking into the department around 7 AM, stating with a subtle smile, "Well Sherry, how's she doing? I didn't receive a call." She continued to improve. The rest of the story is as they say...her history.

Tansy, I have never been the same. I was touched. The days to follow, as you know best, were challenging. Your strength, determination, maybe even a bit of sass; all inspiring.

Thank you for being you, for paying it forward, and simply being present. You are a blessing! God is Good!

Your friend and Nurse,
Sherry

After all those years, I still have the Steno Book my dad is referring to here. It was a small 6 by 9 inch spiral bound notebook that many of my friends, family and some health care workers wrote messages in. I'll share some of their entries here.

Sweet,

I was watching a movie in the theater when an usher told me I had a phone call. You gotta come through this, we need you so bad here Hun. You mean so damn much to us. There's something about you that I loved so much, it just made me happy to be around you. You're one of the coolest girls I've ever met, and I need you. I'll see you soon. Love ya.

Josh

Hey Sweet,

Well I decided we should go to a movie so when you get out, we are going to a movie. No fighting it. I love you sooo much.

Brian

Hello Tansy,

We will be here waiting the whole time for you. Just take your time. I got a T.V. out here to watch.

Love,

Camden

Tanny,

As soon as I heard what happened I couldn't believe it and didn't want to. I wanted to drive up to Neenah right away. I knew I had to see you. I love you so much and can't wait to share the rest of each other's lives with each other. Hang in there and know that I will always love you. I will keep praying for you.

Love,

Elisa

Hi Tansy,

Your Grandma and Grandpa Kuchenbecker have been here to see you each day and night. We think of you all the time and pray for your complete recovery. We look forward to having you waiting on us at A&W. All our love from both of us.

Grandma and Grandpa

Tansy,

All our hearts are with you. I can only imagine the personality you hold. You have so many loved ones and friends who clearly care about you and find you special. Your parents are special people as well. I'm praying for you. God is holding you close right now, and he will always keep you near.

Sherry RN

Dear Tansy,

I was on the trauma team the night our helicopter brought you into E.R. I worked on you without knowing who you were at the time. Only later did I hear your name, Tansy Sweet- in shock because I had taken care of a precious one and only Tansy 17 years ago in our neonatal nursery. I remember quizzing your mom about why she chose your name. You were named after a flower! How appropriate that is. You have brought beauty and joy and love into the world...

Love you Hun, even if for a short while our paths crossed again.

Sharon Respiratory Therapist

Sweet,

I saw you today. I couldn't believe how you were doing. I didn't say too much because I didn't want to take away from Brian's time. I hate you for making me lose my breath and almost dropping. You still were beautiful, like always, and I love you so much. Pull through please.

Matt

5:00 AM I called Cindy at her parents' house to request Elisa to come in for Camden. All the Sweets (Randy, Cindy and Elisa) came right over. (Justin is enroute from Chicago via Greyhound Bus).

7:00 AM Dr. Sears (Ortho) puts in fixators to further stabilize Tansy's broken femurs. Julie and I questioned the procedure due to Tansy's setback. Sears checks with Dr. Wasco and goes ahead. (Tansy's legs were in traction prior to this with 20 lb. weights.)

Twenty-three years later, Dr. Sears agreed to share what he remembered from those initial critical days following the crash:

It has been so many years now, but I remember vividly the candid discussions I had with the other members of Tansy's treatment team as she lay in critical condition in the intensive care unit shortly after her accident.

As an orthopedic trauma surgeon, I understood the dangers posed in leaving the bone unstabilized, especially in a multi-injured young adult. Routine nursing care, likewise, was complicated by two unstable extremities.

Tansy was at risk of fat embolism syndrome, a life-threatening condition that results from fatty bone marrow spilling into venous channels within the broken bones, then entering the body's general circulation. The fatty material passes through the heart and directly into the lungs where it occludes arterioles and capillaries, and in some individuals, sets off a severe inflammatory response compromising gas exchange in the lungs. The longer the broken bones remain unstable, the fattier marrow can be shed into the lungs, accumulating to the point where already damaged lungs can no longer function to sustain life.

Temporary repair of the bone was the best option to reduce risk of developing fat embolus syndrome and to aid in routine nursing care. Tansy's condition would not allow for transfer to the operating room to place external fixators, a quick and minimally invasive procedure to temporarily rigidly stabilize the broken femurs. There, X-ray can be used in real time to accurately place heavy pins into the bone through tiny incisions, then optimally align it with externally placed bars and clamps.

After discussion the team quickly agreed to allow bedside placement of the external fixators without the benefit of real time X-ray, a procedure that I have done only a handful of times in my career. Operating room personnel quickly assembled, prepared necessary equipment, and set up for the procedure in the confining spaces of the ICU. The preparedness and efficiency of our trauma support staff was truly admirable, and to this day, remains fondly impressed in my memories. Though the conditions were less than ideal, the procedure took only minutes, and Tansy's condition remained unchanged.

I was able to sleep that night knowing I had done my part to minimize her orthopedic-related risks. Other trauma team members, however, would spend sleepless hours watching over her.

After a number of days, through the efforts of a well-coordinated trauma team and Tansy's strong youthful constitution, she improved enough to undergo definitive surgery to insert stabilizing rods into her femurs. Her story will long be impressed in my memory as emblematic of a well-functioning trauma program with specialized facilities and dedicated medical specialists.

Dr. Sears

> *7:30 AM Dr. Wasco talks with Julie and me about Tansy's condition. Lungs are doing significantly better. Blood pressure has bounced back. Liver function (two pink viable lobes). "She's a fighter. She's a little better than yesterday. Expect ups and downs."*

7:50 AM Debbie Struble, the EMT who attended to Tansy on the highway, arrives to tell her story (no airbag). Tansy was very combative. Pulled out one IV, tore off some monitor patches. Theda Star was dispatched shortly after Clintonville ambulance arrived on the accident scene.

8:30 AM Lisa Olmsted, the other EMT, arrived to visit. She assessed Sarah first. Then went to assist with Tansy after determining Sarah had died. Lisa and Debbie both go in to see Tansy.

This next memory isn't documented in the journal, but it is in the photo album, and it always stuck out to me.

Somewhere during this time frame, my mom and nurse Sherry decided it was time to brush through my hair as it was matted with blood from the crash, tangled and forgotten in the rush to keep me alive.

The photos show the two of them combing through my hair, a pad under my head covered in blood. My mom couldn't change what had happened, but she could do this one thing. Together, they began gently brushing through my hair, strand by strand, washing away the blood that clung to it. I didn't feel it then, but I imagine my mom's hands were shaking, her heart breaking, yet she did it anyway.

I later talked to Sherry about this moment specifically, and it remains a vivid memory for her. She said they finally had a moment free from lifesaving measures, and my mom desperately wanted to brush through my hair. My mom told Sherry she didn't want to cut it. It took a lot of time, effort and conditioner, but they eventually got through it.

In the next photo, my hair is in a nice, neat braid at the top of my pillow. It wasn't just about getting me cleaned up, it was an act of love and dignity. In a moment where everything about me seemed fragile and broken, she found a way to remind herself that I was still me.

> *1:00 PM Many more high school students from Tansy's class came to spend the PM with us. Randy, Cindy, Justin and Elisa were here. Rodney, Nancy and Sarah came a couple times.*
>
> *Nancy went shoe shopping for Cam. His "Soaps" smelled so bad they had to condemn the private waiting room Camden occupied.*
>
> *A mom of one of Cam's friends brought Cody and Kelsey and some of his other buddies to be with Cam. Then Cam went to spend the day/night with Kelsey. We'll pick him up at 3:30 PM tomorrow so he can go with me to Sarah's wake.*

My dad later shared with me that the friends, family and people from Clintonville who came to visit were incredibly supportive. He said he didn't know how we would've gotten through this without them showing up so consistently.

5:30 PM Dinner at Morris'. Julie waits at the hospital, and we bring dinner for her.

6:30 PM Twenty more visitors. I begin to feel like a tour guide. I have got to change that tomorrow. We've told this story a lot today.

I was still in a medically induced coma at this point, so I don't recollect any of this... just the dreams that went on and on... Scenes that made no sense, people who appeared then faded away, moments that felt so real I was sure they had happened. It was like my brain was trying to piece together the story that my wounded body was undergoing.

Day 5

June 16, 2002 Father's Day

2:00 AM Woke up together to go back to see Tansy. The dialysis is working to filter and pull a little fluid so that input=output.

Every hour the amount of intake is different. They keep tweaking it in the meantime.

Tubing has been clotting causing her to lose a little volume in tubing. It means her blood is clotting.

Sherry has her "Jesus loves you bear" in her hand.

We were very scared walking down there tonight. I was so scared I had to sit down and drink orange juice.

It makes my heart hurt that my dad got so scared, emotional and ill-feeling that he had to sit down. My mom was a nurse for a long time, so she did well in situations like this, though I'm sure it's very different when it's your daughter. I admire the strength it took to sit by my side, to stay composed, to keep the faith that I would be okay. And then how they could fall apart the moments that strength gave way, when the weight of it all became too much.

My dad took a photo of me holding a little bear in my hand. In fact, it appears in multiple photos throughout my hospital stay. It was a gift from one of our neighbors.

5:00 AM Julie was up several times during the night checking on Tansy. Sherry said, "She's peeing like a racehorse." She may be trying to get that fluid out of herself now.

A possible complication of such rapid fluid loss is diabetes insipidus. They're monitoring her specific gravity levels. Blood pressure remained good all night long.

7:00 AM Tansy's color looks much, much better on her face, her shoulders, arms, and legs. I noticed her ears are pink and less swollen. Julie thinks Tansy's lips are less puffy, too. (Geddie says Tansy has chicken lips.)

As flattering as it sounds, the nickname I got from several of my guy friends in high school was "bird lips."

Debbie S., Tansy's EMT stopped by earlier this morning to talk. I told her Jason S. called and said Tansy was conscious enough to work the gum up to the front of her mouth so they could get it out.

Both Debbie and Jason said they can't get Tansy off their minds. Prayers keep coming.

Tansy has a fever of 101 degrees Fahrenheit.

7:15 AM Night shift is giving the day shift report. I told nurse Kay that we will cut way back on the visitors so that we're out of their way and lessen the chances of infection.

Nurse Sherry made a sign handwritten in black sharpie on a piece of paper and taped it to the outside of my CCU room door. It read, "Visitors, please stop at Nurses Station. Thank you." The photo of this sign still sits amongst the other memorable photos in the brown album, depicting the silent, chronological version of this story. It goes hand in hand with my dad's journal entries. Both are vital aspects of my emotional healing and recovery to this day.

7:55 AM Julie is at Morris and Jean's showering. Her only daily break- she won't even go down to the cafeteria.

8:30 AM Dr. Wasco said she's continuing to hold her own. Today will be used to get her ready for surgery tomorrow. That will involve unwrapping the liver that is in plastic, cleaning the area, patching it with dissolvable gauze and trying to partially close the opening. It may be too early to do the trach or the feeding tube into the stomach. They will be trying to get some nutrition into her today.

12:00 PM Dad picks me up. We drove to the accident scene on the highway. Some of the kids have set up a memorial to Sarah at the site of her death.

While I was paying my respects to Sarah at the crosses, Dad paced off the length of the skid marks (120-130 feet).

My dad photographed the memorial at the crash site, so I would eventually be able to see it. He also took a photo of my Grandpa Sweet walking along the skid marks on the highway as he measured them with his stride. I'm thankful to my dad for photographing these moments for me.

Next, we drove home and met Cam. He was showering. Several messages were on the answering machine. I picked up a few things, showered and cleaned up after the cats. Geddie was there cutting and trimming the lawn.

9:00 AM I called Sarah's dad and asked permission to photograph Sarah in her coffin. My rationale was I thought Tansy may need to see that someday for validation that Sarah was really gone. He understood but requested I do it before the visitation began.

Sarah's dad was a wonderful man. He treated me like a daughter of his own. We loved him very much.

Sarah's mom passed away during our freshman year of high school. The two of us were pulled out of class together when her dad came to tell her the news. We were only fifteen, just kids ourselves, suddenly facing a kind of grief we barely understood. I sat with her in those early days, not knowing what to say, but knowing she needed me there. We leaned on each other in the way only young best friends can. Neither of us could have imagined that only two years later I'd be the one grieving her.

9:30 AM Dr. Whiteside, the pulmonologist, reports Tansy's lungs are much improved.

Dr. Sears explains to us how he will repair Tansy's broken femurs when the time is right. Titanium rods will be screwed into the bones. No casts will be required, and they'll get Tansy up right away so she can bear weight.

The plan was for bilateral intramedullary nails, a roughly twelve-inch-long rod, that would run the length of both of my femurs. He would make an incision at my knees, insert rods into the medullary cavity of each femur, ream them into place and secure them with screws. I specifically recall hearing him tell me that my femurs could never be broken again while the nails were in place.

> *3:00 PM Dad, Camden, and I arrive at Rhodes and Beil Funeral Home. I took pictures. Tansy's "Best Friends" bouquet of a dozen roses, 10 red and 2 white, are placed next to the head of the casket. Sarah is laid out in orange and black Clintonville Truckers jacket. A baseball signed by her softball team lies in a glove by her waist. She's holding a rosary.*

I'm thankful my dad was able to attend the visitation, pay his respects from our family to hers and see Sarah. I didn't even know she had died at this point, as I was still unaware of what had happened.

My dad carried a double weight, splitting his time by being at my side and representing me at hers. I couldn't go to the visitation. I couldn't say goodbye. I couldn't stand beside everyone else grieving her. I was later told details about the visit by my dad and my friends who were in attendance.

I still have the "best friends" ribbon that was in the bouquet of roses that my parents had sent from me. Sarah also wore her class ring.

We drop Cam off at Cody N's. He'll spend the night there tonight.

5:00 PM We return to Theda Clark with clothes and Tansy's bulletin board of pictures.

During the PM, Julie met with a couple from Red Granite whose daughter had a remarkably similar experience. Her friend died, this 18-year-old suffered a severe liver injury, she was cared for in Tansy's room 109. Ten days have passed and now she's up on the 6th floor recovery unit.

Carpenters came by with stationery, stamps, toiletries and a great idea; a portable CD player with a CD of easy/soothing Christian music. Tawny's listening to it as we speak.

We had a good time talking and laughing. Nancy K. stopped by too with a lot of Avon products.

A little later in the evening, Jack and Carole D. visited following Sarah's wake.

Two kids snuck down the other hallway and were standing at Tansy's doorway. The nurses escorted them out to us just as I was tuning in to watch Brad Spakowitz at 10:15. We visited briefly, then politely told them we were tired at 10:30.

Day 6

June 17, 2002

7:00 AM Tansy's condition continues to improve. Dr. Sears told us that comparing how she was on Wednesday when she was admitted to now, she's doing fantastically.

Dr. Wasco is doing more surgery on Tansy today at about 2:30 PM. He will be unwrapping the plastic surrounding the liver, doing a trach so her mouth and throat can be freed of the NG tube and ET tube, and he may put in a feeding tube if he can close her abdomen a little more. They will also clean the wounds while in surgery.

We pray, Lord, that you will be with Tansy and the doctors and nurses during this surgery. We pray she won't be set back from this, that He will help her to continue to progress on this long recovery.

10:30 AM Sarah's funeral is taking place in Marion now.

While I was lying in the hospital, Sarah was laid out in the church. Her funeral happened without me. That absence is something I'll never forget. Another bit of grief that lives alongside my survival.

I was still in a coma, unaware of what had happened. My parents stayed at the hospital with me, but most of our friends attended Sarah's funeral.

It's something I've had to process over time. While I was fighting for my life, the people I loved were fighting through their grief. My dad showed up for me and Sarah, in a way I never could have at the time.

Brian, Ryan, Josh, Matt, and Geddie were the pallbearers. Kids themselves... One of them shared with me that, at the burial, they all went up to her casket before lowering her into the ground and each took a rose. Brian and Josh eventually gave their roses to me.

June 17th is also the birth date of three of our close friends who were in attendance. Sarah's funeral fell on their golden birthdays.

My good friend Rachel was unable to attend the funeral due to a flight for a family vacation. She shared this with me, "On the way to the Green Bay airport that morning, my dad stopped the car so I could place flowers at the crash site. He felt bad that I couldn't attend her funeral but said to me, 'Just think Rachel, while you're on the plane, you'll be the closest one to heaven and the closest one to her for a while.'"

2:30-5:30 PM Tansy has surgery. She has a trach to which the respirator is now attached, Dr. Wasco unwrapped the plastic from around her liver, put a feeding tube in her belly (temporary) and closed her up completely. No transfusions were needed. She's had over 100 units of blood and blood products since last Wednesday.

One hundred units!!! In less than a week. This was the very beginning of my lifelong journey as a blood donor advocate.

A G-tube, or gastrostomy tube, is placed in the stomach through the abdominal wall and a J-tube, or jejunostomy, tube is placed in part of the small intestine. Both are types of feeding tubes used to deliver nutrition directly to the digestive tract. Once the nursing staff started using my J/G tubes, they needed to flush them routinely. In the days to come, after I became aware of my surroundings, this process would make my belly feel remarkably full.

7:30 PM Heather G. and her family came up to see Tansy and us. She was in a serious car accident 10 days ago. She's 18 with a fractured pelvis, a broken wrist, had a severe liver injury, she was in a drug-induced state of paralysis. She had been on a vent. She had been flown here in the helicopter. Her best friend died in the accident.

I hope Tansy comes through all this like Heather has progressed.

I'm certain that the mutual support that was developed between my parents and Heather's parents gave my mom and dad some hope. She recovered and came out on the other side. They were able to talk, compare stories and share fears. They had a rare, but deep common bond, developed within those hospital walls.

Day 7

June 18, 2002

Tansy developed a blood clot in her right leg extending from her groin to her knee.

An interventional radiologist performed a surgical procedure at 3:00 PM to place a filter called a "Gunther Tulip Vena Cava MReye Filter" in her vena cava to catch the clot should it release. It looks kind of like a badminton birdie.

We bumped into Dr. Georgen in the hall. He's amazed at her progress. No longer is it minute by minute, now it's more like hour by hour, or even day by day.

I was the perfect storm to develop a clot or deep vein thrombosis (DVT): major trauma, several extensive surgeries, long bone fractures, immobilization and birth control. The filter was placed to prevent pulmonary embolism (a clot in the lungs) which would have been a life-threatening complication of its own, if the clot released.

I was unable to use anticoagulants due to the continued risk of hemorrhage from my liver. The blood clot possibly formed due to the pressure utilized to pack my abdomen to stop the hemorrhaging. Fast forward to twenty years from this date, and I had my IVC filter removed by an amazing interventional radiologist in Green Bay.

Day 8

June 19, 2002

Dr. Wasco is concerned about the toes on Tansy's right foot. They may have to be amputated. Dr. Georgen told me the same thing.

This may have been the first time my parents were informed I would lose the toes on my right foot. My parents told me later, and nurse Sherry told me recently (as we have become friends), that it was possible I could've lost all my fingers and toes due to compromised circulation from the medication given while I was in critical condition.

Dr. Georgen also showed me the X-rays of her vena cava filter and the food tube going into her stomach and small intestine. They're going to start giving her nutrition through there soon.

Dr. Sears said he may be fixing her femurs a week from yesterday- which would be on Tuesday, June 25th.

Georgen said again all her vital signs are looking miraculously better.

There are photos partially showing my legs. Both of my knees had bruises from hitting the dash-board, resulting in bilateral femur fractures. My dad never got a photo of the toes on my right foot, but there is a photo showing the toes on my left foot, and they looked like they were in bad shape too. They were very deep red in color.

My body was in survival mode. To keep my vital organs perfused, I was given vasopressors, which are medications that constrict blood vessels to raise blood pressure. These drugs prioritize blood flow to the heart and other vital organs, often at the expense of the fingers, toes and limbs.

Sherry later told me that my fingers had also turned a dark red color. Luckily, all my fingers and the toes on my left foot rebounded and regained circulation. However, the toes on my left foot have never been the same since. They are scarred, very sensitive and get cold easily in the winter.

11:00 AM Dr. M. takes Tansy off the paralytic medication.

1:00 PM Renee G. came by and sang an inspirational song for us. Nancy K. was here too.

Jon Hagen, her flight nurse, introduced us to the other flight nurse, Ann Younger. He gave me this information on the Theda Star flight:

June 12, 2002
Accident: 4:18 PM
Call came in: 4:27 PM
Lift off AMC: 4:33 PM

Gas stop at Maxair: 4:37 PM
Departed Maxair: 4:39 PM
Arrived on scene: 4:53 PM
Left scene: 5:19 PM
Arrived at TC: 5:37 PM
Total: 1 hour 10 minutes

6:05 PM Tansy is still resting comfortably. Very stable. No signs of coming out of the coma have been seen yet. It may take several days. Tansy's toes on her right foot don't look good.

8:00 PM Heather G. stops by for another visit.

Day 9

June 20, 2002

6:50 AM I'm sitting on the floor in Tansy's room listening to the rhythmic sound of the ventilator. Tansy is still in critical condition. Her vital signs have remained good through the night.

Dr. Sears just stopped in and looked at her toes on her right foot. He said the toes aren't looking good, but the rest of them are hanging in there. The surgery on her femurs is still scheduled for next Thursday, June 25th if things continue to go as planned.

Today they're going to try Tansy on a blood thinning medication called Lovenox. It will be a shot injected into her belly area, I guess. We pray it will keep her from developing any more blood clots while also not causing her to bleed. (They'll be watching her closely.)

The paralytic agent was stopped yesterday. Today Dr. Wasco cut her Versed in half. She's still on Morphine.

10:05 AM Julie went home to Clintonville to take care of business quickly and come back.

I saw Tansy's incision today for the first time. What a trauma she has had to endure!

I'm sure the first time my dad saw my abdominal incision was overwhelming for him. My body had been cut open from my breastbone to my pubic bone, a long, raw reminder of how close I had come to death. He already knew what the surgeons did, but words couldn't prepare him for seeing it with his own eyes.

My incision wasn't the typical thin, straight line closed with sutures or staples. It was a long, jagged cut left gaping open to heal by secondary intention, from the inside out.

My abdomen looked like a war zone, and he could see all the layers. Yellow subcutaneous fat. My belly button tilted on its side. Large raw areas, scabbed areas and tissue in various stages of healing. Surgical pen markings on my skin in the places that hadn't yet been damaged from tape. He saw it all.

I would imagine he caught a glimpse during a bandage change while I was still in the coma. I didn't allow anyone other than nurses and my mom to see it for several weeks after I woke up. I was very self-conscious about it at first as I felt very open and exposed.

> *Michelle K., the school nurse, just called inquiring about Tansy's condition, and I filled her in.*
>
> *She's going to Rock Island this weekend. I asked her to make sure she gets a tour of the lighthouse. I also asked her to let people know about Tansy's condition and to pray for her.*
>
> *Michelle wondered if there was anything she wanted me to do for Tansy while she was there. I asked her to pick the prettiest flower she could find on her hike to the lighthouse and to lay it on the lantern and say a prayer for Tansy.*
>
> *Met helicopter pilot Tim L. He was the pilot on Tansy's flight. He showed Camden, Drew and me the choppers.*
>
> *10:40 AM TANSY OPENED HER EYES FOR ME!!!*

When I finally opened my eyes after waking up from the coma, the first person I saw was my dad. My vision was foggy and shapes blended together. It felt like I was looking through water. I struggled to focus and was unsure of what was real. I wasn't sure I was even awake, or if this was still some form of altered reality like in my dreams. But in the end, it was my dad's face that came into focus.

My dad was standing at my bedside wearing a tie. At least in my memory. The more I think about it, he probably wasn't in a tie while living in the CCU in the hospital for the past nine days.

I couldn't speak. I didn't understand what had happened or where I was. But opening my eyes and seeing him there next to me grounded me. That blurry, memorable moment was the beginning of finding my way back.

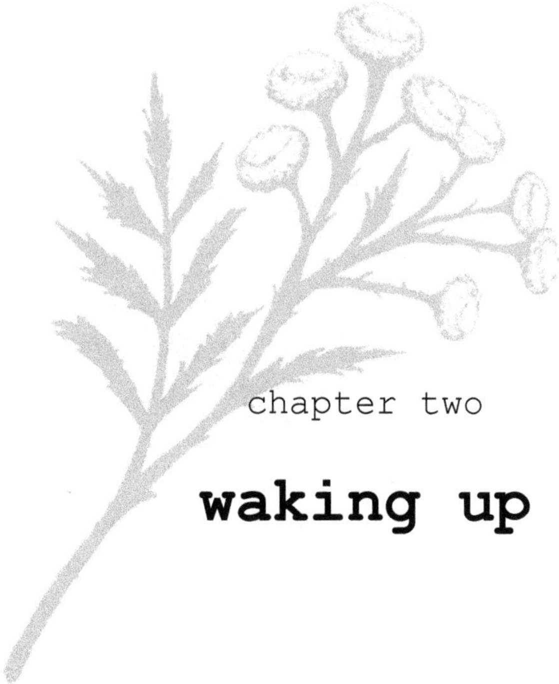

chapter two

waking up

Day 10

Friday, June 21, 2002

8:50 AM Tansy is continuing to come out of her drug-induced paralysis.

We stayed up with her all night trying to comfort her. She's unsure of where she is so we continue to remind her.

She will be unable to talk while the trach is in place. We're telling her that, too.

She has nodded "no" to Julie's question about listening to music. And she nodded "yes" to nurse Kim when she was talking to her.

She grimaces when we tell her she's in the hospital.

The nurses and doctors told me I was "very sick." This was confusing because I didn't feel sick. I felt hurt. I was badly injured in a car crash; I was perfectly healthy before that. I had no idea how sick I was.

> *9:30 AM Dr. M., a pulmonologist detected pneumonia in Tansy's lungs. That is a common side effect of being on a respirator for extended periods of time. He's treating it. Also, they're trying to slowly wean her off the ventilator so that she can breathe on her own.*
>
> *10:10 AM Dr. Wasco tells us he's going to Las Vegas for a week to a surgical convention. Dr. Burkett and Dr. Georgen will be taking care of Tansy while he's gone. He'll check in on her periodically via phone.*
>
> *He said when she came in, Tansy had about a 1% chance of living through this. Then it progressed to 30%. Now he's looking forward to seeing her up on the rehab unit. We are too! We love Dr. Wasco.*

The feeling of gratitude that I have toward the trauma surgeons who saved my life isn't just thankfulness; it's something deeper. Heavier. Sacred even. It's an awareness that in my most broken, vulnerable moment, their hands, determination and decision-making are what stood between me and the end of everything.

Dr. Wasco later wrote a letter to my parents stating, "Working with Tansy has been one of my most gratifying experiences in medicine. I am so proud of how hard she has worked to overcome serious life-threatening illness and subsequent setbacks."

> *3:00 PM We talked to one of the nurses who attended to Tansy in the new ER Trauma Center. Tansy was one of the first critically injured patients to go through there since it opened June 4. She showed me the bed on which they attended to Tansy. She also explained that the rapid infusion machine was used to get four units of blood into Tansy before she went into surgery.*
>
> *They did an ultrasound there to confirm internal bleeding. The digital X-ray machine was not used because it was obvious she had two broken legs. It was critical to get a CT scan (no brain injury was seen) and then get her to the operating room.*

I recall seeing my bilateral femur X-rays for the first time. I had major fractures on both sides. The two biggest bones in my body were broken in two, with my left femur being an open fracture, meaning the bone punctured the skin on the outside of my left thigh. I've got the specific scar sequence there to remember it by.

> *3:15 PM Ginger and a student did physical therapy on Tansy in bed moving both arms,*

hands, and her left leg. They left the right leg alone because of the blood clot.

Tammy (OT) also assessed Tansy today and yesterday.

A nurse practitioner for the neurologist was in to ask Tansy to track things with her eyes, wiggle her fingers and toes, nod her head, and smile.

Our girlie is on the road to recovery.

As I became more alert and aware, I recall reaching down and feeling the external fixators attached to both of my thighs. It was a strange feeling to have metal connected to and coming out of my body.

9:00 PM Tansy shook her head no (emphatically) when Julie asked if she wanted her to leave during her bed bath. When asked if she wanted her to stay, she squeezed her hand.

Tansy mouthed "I love you" to me as I was leaving to go with Cam and Elisa to Grandma and Grandpa's.

She smiled at Elisa and looked into her eyes as if she was saying goodbye.

I distinctly recall that when my cousin Elisa was there, I noticed the photo collages on the walls of my hospital room for the first time. I motioned for her to grab one and bring it over for me to see. I thought she had made them, and I wanted to show interest and appreciation. Of course, they were taped to the walls with what seemed like Gorilla Tape because it took a lot of effort for her to get one down. I admired her for not giving up the struggle for me.

Day 11

June 22, 2002

12:00 Midnight Thunder showers woke me. I couldn't sleep after just 2 ½ hours at the folk's house.

I came back to the hospital at 12:25 AM. Julie and I stay up with Tansy through most of the night.

10:00 AM Camden and Elisa come to see Tansy. She's much more alert and moving her arms and legs more.

Dr. M. assesses her lungs and says they have improved a little since yesterday. (Later we give her water on a sponge and cold popsicles-that sets her lungs back a little.) The trach care/suctioning is hard for us to watch.

Her belly is very painful to her. Morphine is continued IV and boluses when her dressing changes occur.

Having my tracheostomy tube suctioned was uncomfortable. It's done sterile, and I could feel the little cannula going down into my trachea. It tickled and made me cough each time. The sound of a person being suctioned is hard to describe to someone who's never heard it before, but it's loud and sounds wet. Pink saline bullets were squirted into my trach by the nurse or respiratory therapist prior to suctioning to loosen secretions. I thought they tasted sweet.

10:30 AM Camden, Elisa, and I drove to Clintonville to get Cam organized for basketball camp at UWSP.

Elisa helps vacuum. We give the cats some TLC. I dust mop floors and clean bathrooms. Mail and papers are brought in. The flower gardens and grass show a lack of attention. Naughty and his buddies are lonely for human contact. I downloaded more of Tansy's photos onto the computer.

Julie stays with Tansy. Randy and Cindy, Rodney and Nancy, Morris and Jean stop by to visit.

"Naughty and his buddies" were a few of our cats at the time: Sassy, Sonny, Morris and Naughty. There were others here and there, but those were the main cats of the household. My mom was a lover of animals, and we had various types of creatures growing up. I'm glad she instilled that in my brother and me.

5:00 PM Julie and I catch a nap while Elisa sits with Tansy.

I picked up supper from the cafeteria, but Julie eats almost none of it. She has me concerned.

It's so hard to see our girl in pain. She also has a fever of about 100 degrees Fahrenheit.

6:00 PM Dr. A., the nephrologist stops in to meet Tansy. She was her kidney specialist. Her services are no longer needed.

9:00 PM Tansy's fever is 101 degrees Fahrenheit. She's still a very sick girl.

Please. God, help her to have a restful, pain-free night.

Julie and I are running on fumes. This isn't easy for any of us. It's so hard to see our girl in pain- struggling to communicate with that trach. But she is such a good patient. What a rocky road she has been through. We ask God to continue to give us all the strength we need to weather this storm.

I bet I was an awful patient, to be honest. I was a 17-year-old who just had her life shattered overnight.

The difficulty with communication on my end due to the trach didn't help things. I was unable to respond verbally, so my only options were either nodding my head "yes" or "no" or scribbling an answer on a dry erase board.

I didn't feel well. I was in pain, physically and emotionally. I wasn't happy. I didn't feel like participating in cares. I didn't feel like answering questions from doctors and therapists. I was grieving my old life while fighting for a new one. And at this point I didn't even know the worst of it.

10:00 PM Nurse Mary told us both to go and get some sleep. We're glad to have that direction.

Day 12

June 23, 2002

4:45 AM Tansy's air bed is moving her all over the place. She doesn't like the repositioning, but it's supposed to help get her lung secretions loosened, and it should help to prevent bed sores on her backside. The night was a restless one for her.

Christine, her nurse, said it was okay to give her a little water on a sponge or popsicle. Tansy loved that. Then they said it wasn't good and was causing her lungs to get "rattly".

The specialized bed was difficult to get used to and uncomfortable while trying to rest with several injuries. It was almost constantly repositioning me, making a windup noise, and transferred my body weight to help prevent pressure sores. Prior to having this bed, I ended up with a large pressure area to the back of my head. I still don't have hair in that spot today.

> *6:36 AM Julie looks tired. We really must start getting more rest and maybe a little time away from the tense environment of the CCU.*
>
> *A sunny day has dawned. The whitewater continues to rush over the spillway. The heron has returned to the fence to patiently wait for a fish and to keep watch over our Tansy.*
>
> *Keep strong, girlie- God is with you. It's a new day- you're that much stronger than yesterday. It's a miracle you've made it this far. You're over the hump. Keep the faith. We love you. Let the power of prayer and the gentle sound of Enya soothe your tired body.*

My dad is such a good writer. It makes me love him so much reading his entries and feeling his emotions during the most difficult time in our lives.

I've seen a photo of this heron that was frequently outside my window, and my parents later told me about it. This tall, quiet bird kept vigil near the water's edge. To them it wasn't just a heron; it was a sign, a presence to mirror their own long hours of waiting and watching over me. Even though I never saw it myself, the image has stayed with me.

My parents were such nature lovers. I'm sure it brought them some small piece of comfort seeing him there day after day.

10:30 AM Julie has lost 15 pounds in the last 11 days that we've lived at the hospital. That's not saying a whole lot about the caféteria food. I, on the other hand, have bulked up to a plump 185 lbs.

1:00 PM OT is working with Tansy on moving her arms. Then she asked her to write on her whiteboard with a marker.

OT asked- "Are you happy or sad?"

Tansy drew a sad face and wrote- "Sad".

OT asked- "What would make you happy?"

Tansy wrote- "Friends."

OT asked- "Is there a special friend you'd like to see?"

Tansy wrote- "Sarah."

Dr. B., the psychologist here, told us to answer her questions specifically. When she's ready to know the answers to the question of what happened to Sarah, she'll ask. I think Tansy may already have an idea about that.

At that point, I had no idea that the reason I was in the hospital, and the reason Sarah was not, were related. I was waiting for her to show up like she always did.

2:00 PM Camden is registering for basketball camp at UW Stevens Point. His friend's parents are bringing them both. The three days away will be a good distraction for him.

4:00 PM Tansy asked for the writing board. She wanted to know what happened.

We said, "You were in a car accident."

Tansy- "With who?"

Us- "Sarah."

Tansy- "When?"

Us- "June 12."

Tansy- "Who was driving?"

Us- "You were Tansy."

Tansy- "Whose car?"

Us- "Sarah's car."

Tansy- "Is the car okay?"

Us- "No, Tansy."

Tansy- "Is she?"

Us- "No, Tansy. Sarah died in the accident."

Reading this conversation back still gives me chills and makes my heart stop. At that moment, time seemed to have ceased. The room felt quiet and heavy. I stared at my parents, trying to make sense of what I had just been told. It felt like the end of the world in my 17-year-old mind. It felt like the air had been ripped out of the room. Feelings of life and loss collided in me all at once. I was alive, but she wasn't.

I stopped listening. I spiraled into my own mind. I stared off into the distance, focusing on my own thoughts. How could this be happening?

I was trying to heal from my own injuries while also trying to understand how someone so close to me could be gone forever. Sarah. Gone forever.

> *Now the story is out, and Tansy can start to deal with what happened.*
>
> *5:30 PM KC came by to talk to us and to pray with us. He has been offering very good advice and support all along the way.*

KC ended up being one of the people I stayed in touch with after my hospital stay. He helped get my parents and me through this ordeal. Later in life, I asked him several times if he'd be the pastor at my wedding.

> *7:00 PM Tansy asked for Brian to come. He brought Matt and Becca.*

I have a photo from this very moment. This was the first time I was awake with visitors other than my parents and nursing staff. The room felt different the second they walked in. All three of them were standing at my bedside. I was so happy to see them but didn't know how to show it.

Communication was a big barrier for me due to my trach tube and inability to talk. Brian stood to my right and held my hand. Matt was next to him and Bec was on the other side of my bed to my left. I wondered to myself if they blamed me for Sarah's death. But at that moment, their presence mattered more than anything. They talked to me like I was still me, and I was reminded that life outside those hospital walls still existed.

Tomorrow more friends will come for very short visits. Charlotte T. will coordinate this.

9:00 PM Tansy has had so many interruptions and so much nursing care that she is exhausted. While having trach care she was in obvious distress. The nurse tells us to leave so she can fall asleep.

Day 13

June 24, 2002

12:00 Midnight Nurse Lynne wakes us up. Tansy wants to see us. She asks questions about when the funeral was and what it was like. Then Julie and I go back to bed.

My parents were the best support system through all of this. I can't help but be amazed at the emotional strength they showed. They were there the entire time. If they weren't physically in my room, they were in the waiting room. I could ask someone to get them, and they'd come.

My parents were watching their child fight for their life, facing one surgery and setback after the other. I know the incredible strength it took for my mom and dad to face those days. They held onto me while grieving Sarah, staying strong in front of me but breaking down when the weight became too much.

My mom later told me that neither her nor my dad ever broke down emotionally at the same time. If my mom was having a hard day, my dad would be strong. If my dad was breaking down, my mom was his rock. I know it wasn't easy for them. I know there were moments when they broke down in private, but I never saw either one of them cry in front of me during that time. In front of me, they were my steady ground. Their love and constant support reminded me that I wasn't fighting alone.

I've since been told by numerous people and healthcare staff about the unwavering support my parents showed during my hospitalization. It wasn't just noticed in the moment; it has left a lasting imprint.

All of these "conversations" that I had during this time were written on the dry erase board or note pad while my parents talked to me. My handwriting was awful. My dad took a photo of one of these specific whiteboard conversations that was memorable to him.

Prior to the crash, Brian and several of his friends had planned to take a trip to Canada around this time. I wrote the following to my mom during one of our talks, "Brian isn't going on his big vacation to Canada with his buddies because he's not leaving me. I thought that was nice. And

- I don't know what I'd do without you and dad constantly here. I love you."

7:00 AM Dr. Sears has Tansy's surgery scheduled for 4:00 PM tomorrow to fix her broken legs.

9:40 AM Tansy is taken off the ventilator. They're going to try this for three hours at a time. So now she's totally breathing on her own. A hose with humidified oxygen is attached. Tansy is coughing up some secretions.

1:00 PM Charlotte T. coordinates Tansy's visitors. Josh, Alicia and Nathan come for a 5-minute visit.

Tansy has a much more restful day.

7:00 PM Brian, Sarah D. and Lisa N. visit.

I've got photos of several of these visits. My friends were all amazing. Once I was home, Lisa told me that, during one of her visits, she held her breath the entire time so she wouldn't pass her germs onto me.

Day 14

June 25, 2002

Nurse Mary wakes us up saying Tansy wants us. Her temp was up a bit, so we worked at cooling her down.

3:30 AM We say goodnight and go back to bed.

7:30 AM Tansy goes in for a CT scan to make sure she's healing okay and there are no leaks.

Surgery to repair Tansy's two broken femurs is scheduled for 3:00 PM today. Tansy is feeling scared, but she is really such a brave, tough patient. We love her more every day.

I recall going to CT with the external fixators in place and cringing at the thought of having to be transferred off my bed and onto the CT table. The staff that did this transfer were amazing, and it didn't hurt at all. I thought they must be strong and really know what they were doing to have done that without any pain on my end.

8:53 AM Back from the CT scan. Requesting as much water from the ice water sponges as we can give her. The CT scan is all clear. Tansy's surgery is now scheduled for 3:00 PM.

Have you ever had to stay in the hospital with a limit placed on your intake? Those water-soaked sponges were EVERYTHING to me. The ones that had been soaking for a while were better than the fresh ones. They held more water and were more satisfying.

12:30 PM The waiting game is on. Tansy is watching MTV for the first time.

3:30 PM The OR techs picked up Tansy for her femur surgery.

3:45 PM Dr. Sears, the orthopedic surgeon, stops by to say surgery will last about 2 hours. Perhaps a little less time.

5:00 PM A nurse calls the waiting room to say the surgery went well and they were putting in the last screw.

5:25 PM Tansy is back recovering in her room.

5:40 PM Dr. Sears said everything went well. Titanium rods were inserted through incisions by the knee. Then tapped up through the bone and held in place with screws.

When the compound fracture occurred on the left leg, she may need another surgery somewhere down the road because of the small piece that broke in between the two larger pieces of bone. Dr. Sears mentioned a bone graft.

Tansy was in excruciating pain after the anesthesia wore off. They had to push extra morphine to make her comfortable and asleep.

This is another vivid memory. After the surgery, I recovered in my room. I was in incredible pain. Between the anesthesia wearing off and the pain medication I was given, I was having a hallucination that I was taking a test, and there were numbers on the ceiling. I was tasked with sorting these numbers with my fingers and getting them into the correct spots. It probably looked like I was typing on a keyboard or using sign language. Everyone who noticed likely thought I had completely lost it.

I had a PCA pump, or patient-controlled analgesia, which was an IV pump with morphine in it. It delivered a dose of pain medication through my IV at regular intervals, but I was also able to push a button to receive an extra dose, if needed. It was set to only deliver so much medication per hour, so I could never give myself too much.

I pushed the button frantically at times when the pain was unbearable. At the end of each shift, the nurse would document the amount of pain medication received versus the number of times I pushed the button.

10:10 PM Temp is on the rise. Ice packs under her armpits are in place to try to cool her down.

Dr. Georgen ordered 325 mg of Tylenol. Can't give a larger dose because that could be toxic to her liver.

Tonight looks like a long night. Julie is taking the first shift. I'll relieve her in a few hours. Poor Tawny- she sure has been put through the wringer these past two weeks.

11:50 PM Julie has got a major adrenaline rush going. She's fighting to keep Tansy's temp down with ice packs in her armpits, behind her neck, and cool cloths all over. She's doing it!

Tansy is more comfortable, and her pain level is tolerable. She's writing messages telling her mother to "sit" and then saying "I'd like to see the babies" at the hospital when we can push her around. Thank you, God, for continuing to save our girl for us!

I must've been feeling pretty decent (or been high on meds) if I was talking about babies. Sarah used to babysit for a friend's baby, and I would frequently be over during those times. We both loved babies. Seeing TV shows of women having babies in the hospital and the babies in a nursery made me think there was a similar nursery in my hospital. I pictured myself looking through the glass windows of this nursery and watching the little babies all lined up in their bassinets. Sarah would've loved it.

Day 15

June 26, 2002

4:30 AM Julie finally agreed to go to bed. She kept battling Tansy's fever all night long with ice packs and cool cloths.

Mary Beth was Tansy's nurse.

7:00 AM Dr. Sears' nurse checks on Tansy. Circulation to the toes on her right foot continues to improve the color of her toes.

Tansy says, "I want to go home."

It will be a while. Today marks the real beginning of rehab. We'll see if she's able to get into a cardiac chair and out of bed for the first time. Dr. Georgen said the sooner they get her moving, the better.

8-11:00 AM Julie dashed home to Clintonville to take care of a few things and to bring Camden back for a visit.

Tansy got a bed bath, dressing changes, the whole nine yards. She's off the vent and resting now.

An infection control doctor told me there is no specific cause of her temp. It's probably a result of the liver healing or the body trying to resolve the blood clot.

The bandage changes were such a frequent part of my hospitalization, that I can distinctly recall the cold water dripping down my sides while the nurse was packing my incision. Some nurses left the packing too wet, causing those drippings, and others squeezed out the excess water.

Nurse Christine said they're going to get Tansy out of bed later and possibly outside (at the end of the hall)! That would be wonderful. She's really looking stronger today. Tawny is our miracle girl!

12:30 PM Tansy gets out of bed for the first time in 15 days!

1:30 PM Tansy goes outside for the first time, too! It took about six of us to get her down the hall and out the door.

Every single bit of this was quite the ordeal. The number of tubes coming out of me and my inability to help made this a big challenge for everyone involved. I didn't do anything miraculous here. The nurses did the work and transferred me into a cardiac chair which was flat for the initial transfer. Once they carefully slid me over from the bed, they moved the chair into a semi-reclined upright position.

Mission "out of bed" was successful, and they somehow managed to push me outside through a narrow hall with the bulky cardiac chair, oxygen tank and likely several IV pumps. I made it outdoors, along a railing with the river somewhere on the other side. The wind blew air into my trach and kept taking my breath away. I've got a photo of this event with my nurse Christine, my dad, mom and Cam.

Day 16

June 27, 2002

6:00 AM Julie and I slept in the waiting room. Julie got up at 3:00 AM to check on Tawny. The nurses were working with her to control a fever that got up to 102 degrees Fahrenheit.

Lung secretions continue to loosen and she's able to cough those out through the trach.

I called Sarah's dad and he's coming to see her tomorrow.

10:00 AM Poor Tansy is being poked like a pin cushion to get a new IV site going.

10:30 AM Grandpa Sweet pays a visit.

1:00 PM Several friends come to visit- Bricco's, Brian, Dave, Lisa, Amy, among others. (Visit Autumn in room 675).

Autumn was in a car crash March 22, 2002, and ended up with a spinal cord injury at the T8-T9 level. We were eventually introduced while in the hospital at the same time, towards the end of my hospitalization. She was in the hospital doing rigorous outpatient physical therapy on the 6th floor rehab unit.

4:00 PM No luck getting IVs started- Infectious disease says let's try something different.

6:30 PM Three more friends, the girls who were in a different accident on the same highway, pay a return visit to Tansy.

7:30 PM Tansy goes for a stroll in the hospital gardens. Also gets wheeled through the CCU and the nurses' station.

I've got a photo of my mom, Sharon, Sherry and me in the garden. My dad was also there as he took this photo. This may have been the first time I was ever in the garden. It's a beautiful, peaceful place, and I can see why my parents liked going there to regroup and pray. I watched the sky, squinted in the sunlight and felt the breeze without it taking my breath away like it did when I was out by the river.

I'm so thankful my dad took photos of every stage of this challenging experience. I've been back to this garden on a few occasions, and it remains a special place to visit.

9:00 PM Back to bed for the night.

Day 17

June 28, 2002

1:00 AM Sherry wakes up Julie- Tansy wants her mom. Julie helps Tansy get settled again- then sleeps on the La-Z-Boy.

Sherry was a great nurse. She frequently helped me. I was an emotional wreck at times, just wanting my mom, and Sherry got her for me. I loved that. Sherry and I are still in touch today. She's an amazing friend.

Sherry recently informed me that, at one point, I was holding my breath to get the vent to signal an alarm. She told me she came into my room for an alarming ventilator on several occasions, but when she checked on me, everything was fine. At times it appeared I was sleeping. She eventually caught on and asked me if I was doing it on purpose. I nodded yes with a little smirk.

Along these same lines, I talked to Jon about what I remembered from my hospital stay. In 2010 I told him that I recalled holding my breath to see if I could make the machines alarm.

3:30-4:10 AM I go to check on the girls- both are asleep in Tansy's room.

6:00 AM Julie's back to the waiting room love seat. I go to sit with Tawny. Wondering if tonight we'll have different sleeping arrangements if Tansy gets moved upstairs. Thinking it would be nice to get Camden in his own bed for a night. The last 17 days have been far from normal.

Tansy is still a very sick girl who needs a lot of nursing care. This rehabilitation is going to be a long process- it helps, though, when we see the progress being made.

Last night we met a girl from Shawano. She's a 19-year-old accident victim who would like to visit with Tansy today.

Julie loves Sharon, the respiratory therapist. She has a great sense of humor.

I love Sharon, too. She is an amazing writer and sends us a yearly handwritten Christmas card, an anniversary card and each of my kids a birthday card. When I first told her I was writing a book about my experience, I asked her if she'd be willing to write something for me to add. It was mailed to me, handwritten on a tiny Holland America Line note pad that's about 3 by 4 inches:

It is an honor and a privilege to be asked by Tansy to pen a few lines as she authors a book, quite an impressive undertaking but not surprising when it comes to Tansy.

I first met Tansy when she was still in a bassinet at Theda Clark Hospital. Her mother Julie, a friend and nurse co-worker, was looking down at her and I just had to question how the name Tansy was chosen. Her mom, a lover of nature, explained to me that it was a wildflower. After looking it up, I realized that it was not just a pretty yellow flower but was known for its toughness and intimidating nature. It even was labeled as aggressive in some areas. Tansy probably doesn't know I saw her at birth, and I wouldn't know until years later how those qualities would sustain her.

As the years went by for me on staff at Theda Clark, I lost touch with Julie and never thought too much about it until one fateful night when I was on duty and assigned the Trauma Blue team beeper. We heard the loudspeaker announce an incoming critical patient. As a member of the team, I drop everything and rush to the ER to take my place at the head of the bed, assisting in airway management. We don't always know the victim's name because we just immediately begin life saving measures. As I looked at this beautiful teenager with life-threatening injuries, a name finally was announced, Tansy Sweet from Clintonville. A parent's worst nightmare has just been presented to us. It's our job to give this person every opportunity to survive. Later as I found Tansy's parents in the waiting room, I wanted to talk with them and give them hope. It was a challenging case and many setbacks and moments on the cusp of death, but that determined wildflower fought her way to survival. None of it was easy on that long journey but we tried to get her through the dark times by wheelchair rides outside and other distractions. We could only do so much, but the real effort had to come from within Tansy.

I've seen it time and time again like when Tansy's mom died unexpectedly at age 53. There was Tansy with poise, grace and determination to honor her mom despite the grief she was feeling.

Tansy's life hasn't been easy, but she has not shied away from any of it. She's an entrepreneur always looking for more challenges, as if motherhood to three beautiful children wouldn't be plenty to juggle.

She can do anything she puts her mind to, and I will always be her cheerleader. This book is just one more example of her capabilities. She's come so far since that day the Trauma Blue call put me back in her life.

Sharon Auden

11:00 AM Accident report arrives in the mail from Waupaca County Sherrif's Department.

6:30 PM Sarah's dad pays a visit to Tansy for the first time since the accident occurs. He reassured her that he doesn't hold Tansy responsible for Sarah's death.

I vividly recall Sarah's dad standing next to my hospital bed. I could hardly breathe. His daughter was gone, and I was still here.

He held my hand while we talked about Sarah. He told me in his deep, gruff voice that he didn't blame me for Sarah's death. Those words didn't magically take away my grief, but they shifted something inside me. They gave me room to breathe again. The relief I felt to hear him say those words immediately brought a lump to my throat and tears to my eyes. Crying with a trach in place is a different experience. I didn't make a sound. I couldn't. My body was racked with silent sobs. He cried with me and told me to come over to his house anytime like I always used to. He said I'm always welcome. I wrote the 4-digit garage code to his place as a way of saying "I'll be there". This brought a smile to his face.

9:00 PM Tansy's miserable- her Foley catheter had to be redone; she has a yeast infection and her period. They have her back on morphine and a PCA pump. She's tired and didn't get out of bed today.

Day 18

June 29, 2002

12:01 AM Another young accident victim who's been in the CCU recently died overnight.

3:00 AM Julie has a hip pointer from sleeping on a love seat for the last 17 nights. She gets up to check on Tansy, then falls asleep watching TV in the waiting room.

6:00 AM We both get up to sit by Tawny. Her temp is 100 degrees Fahrenheit.

7:00 AM Julie's at her folks taking a shower. Tansy is having her dressing changed. Nurse Jessica wants to get Tansy up twice before 3:00 PM.

I just got caught up on thank you notes.

10:20 PM Dr. Georgen has Tansy go in for a procedure to determine where exactly she is leaking bile. Once they make that determination, then they will decide on how to fix it.

He also said that they are going to have to amputate part of her right foot at some time.

10:30 AM Randy, Cindy and Elisa come to visit. Justin is on Rock Island attending the FORI annual meeting.

12:45 PM Tansy returns from the bile check. The nurses get her out of bed and into a chair. They assist her in standing for the first time. It is very painful and scary. She is coughing lots of secretions out of her lungs through her trach opening.

Standing for the first time in eighteen days after spending the previous two-plus-weeks mostly horizontal was terrifying and difficult. It took a team of knowledgeable and well-trained nurses and therapists to get me seated on the side of the bed. I still had several IVs, drains and tubes coming out of my body from various locations. Each of those people had to help protect and move the tubes with me as I moved.

The change in position made my head feel light and dizzy. I felt weak and helpless. They wrapped me in a gait belt (under my arms and around my chest), so they could also hold onto me. I stood up with a walker to help brace myself, and we were able to get into a mostly upright position. I bet I stood for three seconds. It wasn't graceful, it wasn't for long, but it was a small victory.

> *1:30 PM A speech therapist evaluates her swallowing. He decides to stick with clear liquids at this point.*
>
> *He tried a one-way valve over the trach opening so she could speak. It hurt her and would clog up as soon as she coughed up some secretions. I wish that trach could come out soon.*

Speech therapy was rough. It seemed simple enough. I needed to swallow without aspirating or choking and manipulate fluid around my mouth to get it where it needed to go. But nothing worked quite right.

Attempting to use the speaking valve with speech therapy for the first time wasn't easy either. Perhaps it was too soon. The cap covering my trach tube blocked air flow and made me panic because breathing felt different. This caused me to cough, which immediately plugged the valve with tracheal secretions. Later in my recovery, I was able to speak with this valve after they downsized my trach tube.

2:00 PM Julie is picking up Camden so he can spend a few days with us.

7:00 PM Camden is playing video games on a Play Station 2 that Julie rented for him from Block Buster for the next eight days.

Matt and Brian came to visit, along with some other friends.

8:45 PM I went to sleep at my parents' house. Julie and Cam slept at the hospital.

chapter three

upright

Day 19

June 30, 2002

8:27 AM I got back to Theda Clark about two hours ago. Camden was still asleep; Julie was out praying in the garden. Tansy had a pretty good night, I think.

The Dr. said her lungs are continuing to slowly improve. The fluid in there will be absorbed into the body. I guess the bile test yesterday didn't give any clear answers, so they'll have to try another approach.

Five more patients have been admitted to the CCU since I left last night.

9:15 AM The physical therapist, Nurse Jessica, and the respiratory therapist just had Tansy standing up in a walker twice. It was majorly painful for Tansy. When she struggles it causes her to cough up more secretions from her lungs. I feel so bad for her having to endure such struggles.

Several times a day, I was expected to stand at the bedside with help. It still took a lot of work and effort to get from a laying position to sitting at the edge of the bed. I was connected to tubes, drains and a catheter, all needing to be repositioned as I moved. I had a trach, and I was connected to a ventilator. I had several IV pumps and feeding tubes.

The healthcare team wanted me to do what I could on my own. I would attempt to get my legs to listen and cooperate, to move to the edge of the bed, but they felt heavy and foreign. It wasn't like I could easily communicate how I was feeling either. I could indicate "yes" or "no" with my head, and that was about it. Writing was not an option, while I used all my strength to keep my body in an upright position. Communication was a daily challenge.

With the change in position and extra movement, new respiratory obstacles were presented as well. Secretions loosened, causing coughing and making the task at hand much more difficult. Think of how hard it is to accomplish something when you're unable to catch your breath.

10:35 AM Holly, an ultrasound tech has been checking Tansy's liver all over for a bile leak. I don't know if she was able to determine the location of the problem, however.

As I type my dad's journal, I can specifically relate his entries to the photos in my album since he literally documented almost everything between journaling and photography. I have a photo of this very moment. Seeing the pictures makes me feel like I can relive the moment in my mind. The covers were pulled back, baring my abdomen which made me feel chilled and exposed.

2:10 PM Tansy has been up in a chair for about an hour. We watched part of a movie, but it just seemed to put both of us to sleep. Julie and Camden are out driving around to get away from the hospital for a while.

5:30 PM Dr. Georgen explains different ways to repair the bile leak in Tansy's liver.

6:30 PM Tawny gets put in a chair and goes for a ride up to the 6th floor with Grandma and Grandpa Sweet, Julie, Nurse Laurie and me. The view of the harbor is peaceful and quite beautiful.

Another distinct memory, mostly thanks to a photo from my dad or perhaps the memorable view from the 6th floor overlooking the helipad. The photo I can think of from this moment shows my fingernails painted red. My mom tried so hard to make me feel normal and pretty.

At the time, the critical care unit was on the first floor of the hospital. The rooms didn't have much of a view. To get me out of those same four confining walls of my hospital room, I was frequently taken on short "trips" to other parts of the hospital. I didn't get there in a traditional wheelchair. Instead, I used what they referred to as a cardiac chair. It was a chair on wheels that could convert from being completely flat to a more propped up seated position, like a chair.

I enjoyed being brought up to the 6th floor rehab unit and wheeling down to the south end to look out through the big glass windows. It provided a beautiful view of the sail boats on the water. From there I could see the helicopter hangar and the helipad. Sometimes, Theda Star would be on display after having brought another critical patient to the ER. Other times, it would be taking off or landing. It was always memorable seeing it come and go.

6:50 PM Camden arrives at the hospital in a 1936 Chevy truck. Morris and Jean come for a visit.

8:30 PM Camden and I sleep at Grandma and Grandpa Sweet's house.

Day 20

July 1, 2002

6:00 AM I wake up and get ready to come to the hospital. Grandma will bring Camden later after he gets up.

6:30 AM I stop by Kuchenbecker's to let Abbie out on her spot.

Julie said Tansy threw up last night probably a result of clamping off the stomach tube.

7:07 AM Tansy is napping. She asked for a cool cloth to put on her head.

Dr. Wasco came back to work today.

Julie's down getting some breakfast. She made worry stones to give other family members in the waiting room, and charms for Tansy's caregivers.

My mom was a very artistic and creative person. I can still picture these stones and charms today. She had secured the charm loops to the bottom of an 8" x 10" school photo of me, and it hung on the wall in my hospital room. She gave them to just about everyone who entered my room. The staff hung them from their name tags or stethoscopes.

8:15 AM Dr. Sears was in a short while ago and explained to Tansy that she's going to have to lose the toes on her right foot. He told her how the lack of blood supply and her blood pressure caused the problem. He likened her toes to what happens when a person gets a severe case of frostbite from a winter storm.

He said she should be able to walk normally. Toes are mainly used for balance while standing.

Our girl sure has a lot to deal with.

When I first heard I'd be losing the toes on my right foot, it felt like the ground had been pulled out from under me. Again.

At seventeen, it felt like a devastating loss. My toes looked awful. They were dead and black. They looked like something from a movie, where some poor soul had been lost in the frozen wilderness for days, the unmistakable mark of gangrene setting in after too long exposed to the merciless cold.

Now I was being told a part of me would be gone forever. I didn't know how I would walk again, or if I'd ever feel normal. How would people look at me? What would they think? What would my boyfriend think? I didn't know anyone with an amputation.

I cried and I grieved something most people never even think twice about.

2:00 PM We finished our family counseling session with Dr. B. Camden did not enjoy it. Then I took Cam back to Clintonville.

2:45 PM Tansy goes in for an MRI to try to get more information on her bile leak.

6:00 PM Dr. A. from Oshkosh meets with us. He's not sure the stent will do the trick. The leak most likely is in her bile ducts in the liver. This is a very specialized surgery. Dr. Wasco will consult with one of his mentors, Dr. R. from University Hospital in Madison. More on this latest speed bump later.

7:01 PM Tawny is tired and sleeping. Julie just went to get something to eat.

Cat hair abounds at home. The flower gardens have grown leaps and bounds. Water lilies are blooming. The bittersweet vines look like a jungle gone wild.

8:00 PM Tansy, Julie and I watch "Kate and Leopold" on the VCR. Tawny wrote, "Will you get me an orchid?"

That's my mission today.

This has been an ongoing memory for me and my parents over the past twenty-three years. There was a gorgeous orchid in this random movie we had watched together, and I must've said, "Gosh let's get one of those!" The conversation was memorable enough for my parents to save the very piece of paper it occurred on.

On July 1, 2002, my mom wrote "I love you" on a piece of stationary decorated with flowers and a fuzzy brown bear in the corner. I wrote in my messy handwriting, "Will you get me an orchid?"

I'm sure my parents responded verbally, but my dad eventually wrote, "YES, we will - even if we have to pilfer one from a state park." This was funny because it's something he would never do, but he was expressing the extent he'd go through to grant me this small request. My parents said they would've given me a pony if I'd asked for one.

My grandparents ended up getting me a gorgeous pink moth orchid. I can still picture them walking into my room with it in their hands. There are several photos of this orchid as it adorned and added cheer to my hospital rooms. To this day, I have several orchids in my southern-facing kitchen window. They're symbolic and memorable of this time in my life.

> *Dr. Wasco walked by laughing as I was trying to get the attention of the woman who watches the closed-circuit patient TVs.*
>
> *10:00 PM The movie is over. (Tawny liked it.) Sherry gets Tansy out of bed and into a cardiac chair. We all take a walk down to the ER and through the garden.*
>
> *10:30 PM Dr. Wasco explains it would probably still be a good idea to do the procedure of placing a stent near Tansy's liver. It may provide a path of least resistance and allow the bile to begin flowing through. That could give the other bile ducts a chance to heal on their own. He said we have time because the drain is*

continuing to do its job. He still is going to talk to Dr. R. about his opinion.

Day 21

July 2, 2002

6:00 AM Julie stayed on her love seat all night without having to check on Tawny. We both went to bed last night for the first time feeling a little more at ease.

Tawny was picking the scabs off her blisters on her left hand. That made Julie think she was showing signs of caring about something.

I don't think the reason for the blisters was noted in the journal so let me elaborate. My hands were cold due to reduced blood flow to my periphery, because the vasopressors I was given initially constricted blood vessels to keep vital organs alive. At one point, an IV bag was heated and placed on my hand to warm it. The combination of the warmth and my sensitive skin ended up causing some blisters on my left hand. They were big, but they eventually went away. I have faint scars on my hand from them today.

6:35 AM Julie is catching a shower at her parents. I have three more cards to write out.

1:00 PM Grandma and Grandpa Sweet brought Tansy a beautiful moth orchid to brighten her room. Now we must study how to keep it growing.

I've got a classic photo of this very orchid sitting on the windowsill in my hospital room with a gorgeous view in the background, thanks to my dad's photography skills.

5:00 PM We're waiting for the hospital to find an anesthesiologist to put Tansy to sleep during the bile duct stent procedure. So far, they haven't been able to locate such a doctor. KC talked to Tansy this afternoon. We need to bring in her Bahamas photo album tomorrow.

TV-2 is apparently going to do their Theda Clark Tansy story tomorrow. The hospital PR man has been making the arrangements. They're going to include a Clintonville fund-raising component along with Jon Hagen and the hospital staff that have worked together to save Tansy's life.

7:30 PM Dr. Wasco calls back. He's got another doctor from AMC who will do the procedure sometime between 12:00 and 5:00 PM tomorrow.

9:30 PM I see that Tansy is sad. She starts crying as a nurse and I are wheeling her though 2nd floor. It's probably related to a loss of dignity- she can't talk, she can't walk, she can't pee without a cath, etc. I feel bad for Tansy, too.

Every day there was a wave of different emotions for me. Something would trigger a memory or thought of Sarah, and I'd spiral into guilt that my best friend was gone, and I was alive. Nothing felt fair about that.

My body was broken in ways I couldn't comprehend. I needed constant care and help doing the things I had done alone for years. Pain meds helped blur the edges of reality, but never fully took the pain away. They helped me feel numb. I welcomed that.

Sometimes the grief dug so deep within me, that when mixed with my acute physical pain, I struggled to tell them apart. My body hurt, my heart hurt and my mind was exhausted.

So, I cried.

Day 22

July 3, 2002

2:37 AM I get up to check on Tansy. She's wide awake and asks for juice.

6:00 AM Julie gives me an inspirational article to read given to her by RT Sharon.

Guess what I found nestled inside the inner pocket of my dad's journal!?! This very article. I read it for the first time as I wrote this book, twenty-three years following the crash. The article is deeply moving, and it's called "Recognizing Spirit - Develop Motivation for Healing" by Dr. Lee

Jampolsky. One of his quotes spoke to me; "If you are suffering from the loss of someone close to you, what would that person tell you to do with your suffering?"

As a 17-year-old, I did not quickly move on from the profoundly devastating loss of Sarah. It was hard and healing would take time. Now, as a 40-year-old, Sarah would tell me to live, not just survive. She would tell me to take the trips and hug the people I loved a little tighter. She would remind me that my misery is not a betrayal of her, but an expression of how deeply I loved her. She would want me to transform my suffering into something meaningful. Rebuild it into something that honors her.

This is why I wrote this book.

6:00 AM Julie has a hip pointer.

My parents had so many inside jokes during their marriage. "Hip pointer" was one of them. I can picture my parents laughing about this or something similar in the living room of the home we grew up in.

7:25 AM Waiting for Wasco.

7:35 AM Dr. Wasco tells us this ERCP (endoscopic retrograde cholangiopancreatography) needs to be done whether she goes to Madison or not. It will show exactly where the leak is, which is necessary. Her drain could stay in for six months if it had to. Placement of such a stent will allow establishment of bile flow and facilitate healing.

If it was one of his daughters, he would be totally confident with Dr. D.- a surgeon from AMC.

He's not a second choice. Dr. Wasco always makes us feel better after we talk to him.

9:46 AM PT Ginger puts Tansy on the tilt table for the first time. She was then tilted to an almost vertical position and remained standing for one minute. She then had her knees bent after getting back in bed. The pain was excruciating.

Physical therapy after I had my femurs fixed was painful, but working to regain full flexion and extension of my knees by having them passively bent by another person was torture. However, it was imperative if I was going to regain my range of motion to eventually walk normally, run and do whatever else I wanted. My goal in PT was getting back to climbing the stairs two at a time. This simple goal seemed unattainable at that moment.

10:30 AM Becky and a TV-2 cameraman came to tell the story of all the people (and God) who had a part in saving Tansy's life. They interviewed Julie and me, then Jon Hagen- Tansy's flight nurse, and finally Dr. Wasco, Tansy's other hero.

The tape airs tonight on the 6:00 PM newscast. Julie and I even got a ride in the helicopter.

I briefly knew this was happening, but I didn't witness a single moment of it. The news crew never came into the CCU and never even walked past my room. I'm thankful that my parents sheltered me from the lights and the cameras. It was hard enough to communicate with my family, friends and care team. I was not stable emotionally or mentally to contend with the spotlight or questions from strangers.

In the end, this turned out to be a nice story. Everyone they interviewed did great. The thought of the story of my crash and recovery being on the local news made me feel a little nervous and self-conscious. However, I knew my parents had my best interests at heart and would be sure it was tasteful and accurately portrayed.

After their interview, my parents got to ride on Theda Star. I love that for them. Maybe one day I'll get to ride on it and remember it...

12:51 PM Tansy's ERCP is scheduled for 4:00 PM.

2:43 PM Tammy is Tansy's OT. She really likes her.

My occupational therapist, Tammy, and physical therapist, Ginger, were two people I saw almost every day... sometimes more than daily. At first, it was exhausting just to sit up or move an arm, but they kept showing up for me. They pushed me each day.

PT and OT weren't just about the exercises; they were about rebuilding independence: standing, walking, figuring out how to manage basic everyday tasks again. Their persistence, patience and creativity helped me regain strength and confidence in myself and my abilities.

One of the most creative activities I recall was playing balloon ping pong with foam paddles and a balloon. Tammy introduced it to me for the first time to work on the range of motion in my arms while I was in bed. It forced me to reach up above my head and coordinate the movements of my arms with what I was seeing. It wasn't painful or hard, but lighthearted and less intensive than mundane occupational and physical therapy.

> *3:00 PM Ten of Tansy's good friends meet with the psychologist and speech therapist. Then they come down to cheer Tansy up more than ever before. She's smiling and having a great time with them.*

I've got a photo of this very meeting where my friends met with the medical staff to learn how to best communicate with me. There is also a follow up photo of those same ten friends surrounding my hospital bed afterward.

I wanted so badly to join in the conversation with them. To laugh with them. To say something... anything! Instead, I had to rely on my eyes, hand squeezes and note pads to communicate. It was frustrating for me but also comforting because even in my silence, they still showed up for me.

Those visits meant more than my friends probably realized. They brought pieces of normal life into a place that felt anything but normal. My friends' support meant the world to me.

4:00 PM Michelle comes by for a visit. She has a beautiful letter and pictures for Tansy describing her trip to Rock Island. While she's here, Dr. D. comes to explain the ERCP procedure. We're glad he's the one doing it.

4:10 PM Lena calls. Julie talks to her- then I finish the call so Julie can say goodbye to Tansy before they wheel her off for the procedure.

5:50 PM Dr. D. reports all went well. They cut the sphincter muscle and placed a stent in Tansy's duct near her gallbladder. They could see where the bile was leaking from the left branch of the bile duct. They also received a bile flow through the tube as they had hoped. Now it's time to wait and see if Tansy's liver will heal itself.

6:05 PM Tansy's story airs on WBAY. They put together a great piece- we were pleased and impressed. Three of Tansy's heroes were featured: Jon Hagen, Dr. Wasco and her mother.

I love this so much. My mom, Jon and Dr. Wasco are three of the most memorable people in my life. Other than Sarah, my mom was my best friend.

I hope that the people who watched this news story noticed how strong and composed my parents were. I hope that they felt a stronger bond with my family since we were from such a small community. I hope that others think of their own children and friends and realize how quickly life can change.

7:35 PM Tansy is sleeping off the anesthesia.

Julie is out renting movies and letting Abbie out.

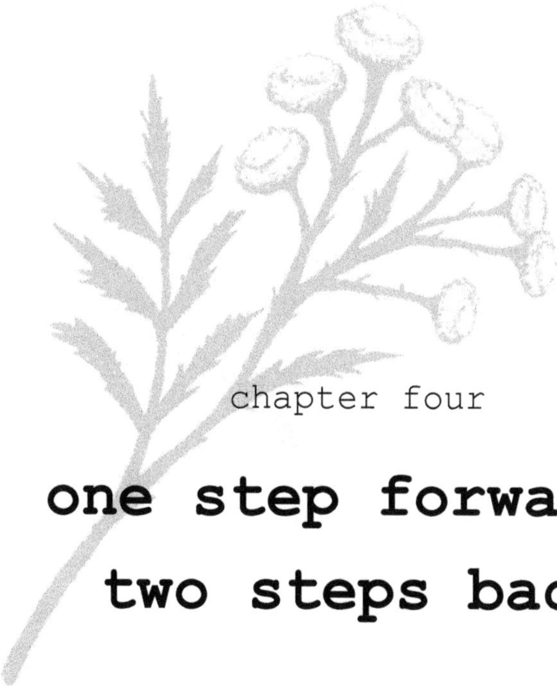

chapter four

one step forward, two steps back

Day 23

July 4, 2002 Independence Day

7:05 AM Dr. Wasco just peeked in on his favorite patient and recapped the ERCP. He, too, said the procedure went well. Then he added, "How'd you like the ride in the helicopter?"

Dr. Wasco is downsizing Tansy's trach. Dr. Wasco said all of Tansy's lab results look good. Her white blood cell count is down. She's moving to the second floor today!

11:30 AM Tansy gets moved out of CCU to the 2nd floor! Now that's a sign of some real progress. We saw Dr. D. a little while ago and he sounded very optimistic about the ERCP.

I was transferred up to the 2nd floor in my hospital bed. The elevator was packed with me in my specialized bed, an IV pole complete with a couple of pumps and two of the CCU nurses who would soon report off to the new nurses taking over my care.

I had grown accustomed to the same group of critical care nurses who had routinely been in and out of my room over the past twenty-three days. They took care of me for over three weeks when I couldn't do a single thing for myself. They kept me alive. I felt apprehensive being in a different environment with different nursing staff. It almost felt like the first day of school. They didn't know me and what I'd been through.

> *The other big news from this AM is that Tansy talked. Since downsizing her trach, when they put the speaking valve on, she could talk. She carried on a conversation with us and even called both sets of grandparents.*

Talking was made possible with a purple valve, called a Passy-Muir speaking valve. I can still picture it very clearly. We kept it in a denture case. It was a little circular cap that slipped over the end of my trach tube and blocked the airflow, so I could speak.

I hadn't said a word in over three weeks at that point. When I uttered my first sounds, I was impressed that my voice worked. I sounded like a quiet, more timid version of myself. I was anxious to show off my newfound skill, so I dialed my grandparent's number to say "hi" and that I loved them. They answered my calls and were so thankful and grateful to hear me talking and using the phone again. Making a phone call, talking and having a conversation were such simple tasks, frequently taken for granted.

I didn't talk for long the first time. It was hard as my vocal cords were weakened from nonuse. It would take practice and time to strengthen them. But it was another small victory for me.

> *2:00 PM PT Amy got Tansy's right leg going on the continuous passive motion machine. It moves slowly.*

The CPM machine is a medical device that moved my knees through range of motion without me having to do anything. At that time, it was more widely used and was a great way to work on ROM without significant pain from manual therapy.

> *8:30 PM Tansy's temp has gone up above 103 degrees Fahrenheit. That's the highest since she's been here. Dr. D. said that it could result from the ERCP (endoscopic retrograde cholangiopancreatography).*

Day 24

July 5, 2002

6:58 AM Tansy and Julie had a rough night. Neither one of them got much sleep. Tansy's temp is still 102.9 degrees, and her heart rate is above 140 beats per minute. We're wondering if this is the result of her ERCP.

Last night I photographed the fireworks from the parking lot and the Oak Street bridge.

This is a vivid memory. I like being warm. I dreamed about being warm and cozy in a room with a fireplace. In my dream, I repeatedly jumped down a flight of stairs onto a pile of pillows. I floated slowly like I was flying and landed softly and gracefully.

Once I awoke from my dream, I realized why I was so warm: I had a high temperature. I didn't have chills frequently associated with a fever. My face was flushed, and I pushed the covers off my arms and torso.

7:59 AM Tansy continues to get treatments from respiratory therapists. Her lungs have been a painful part of this entire hospital stay.

Tawny is dozing, preparing for a busy day. I wish God would slow down her heart rate.

10:30 AM Tansy's white blood cell count is elevated from 17,000 to 43,000. Her temperature is still up at 102.6 degrees Fahrenheit.

The doctors ordered a CT scan of her chest and abdomen. Her lungs are rattly- the coughing really tires her out. This is the shits, God.

I called Camden and told him he might as well stay in Clintonville because of how Tansy is doing.

7:30 PM Shit hit the fan this PM. Dr. Burkett recommended exploratory surgery of her abdomen. Tansy's fever was giving her the chills. Dr. A. ordered ice packs and a cooling blanket. I believe this was just about the longest and scariest day any of us can remember.

Now we wait for Dr. Burkett to finish his surgery marathon until it's Tansy's turn. At the height of the tempest, Pastor H.S. came by. The storm caused him to lose all color in his face. Fortunately, he sat down before he fell. The wait continues as Tansy is now resting more comfortably.

The cooling blanket was dreadful. It's a medical device used to lower a patient's body temperature. It's simply a plastic blanket that goes underneath the patient in bed and cycles cold water through its channels from a cooling unit. The cold water transfers heat from the patient's body to the blanket. I felt chilled from having a fever and was lying on top of a blanket of ice water.

They also had placed ice packs to the back of my neck, my arm pits and my groin to help lower my body temperature. No one would let me have a blanket to cover up with either. Just a sheet. I recall shivering, my body shaking and my teeth chattering.

> *7:58 PM The mom of another patient found Tansy's butterfly balloon and returned it to us when we moved back to 1st floor. I thought it had floated away outside yesterday as we were taking things to the car. They also moved out of our "private suite" in the waiting room and gave it back to us. They didn't have a very good day today either. Some days are like that- especially in the CCU.*

I can still picture this butterfly balloon like it was yesterday. It was a big, colorful mylar balloon in the shape of a butterfly. It was very pretty and girly. It was given to me by four of my girlfriends from school.

Moving back to the critical care unit was a step in the wrong direction and made everything feel uncertain. It was a big setback.

I had already been fighting so hard, and being transferred back to the CCU felt like I was slipping backward into the part of recovery I thought I had left behind. I felt frustrated. I felt angry at my body, scared of what was happening and exhausted from the constant unknowns.

8:50 PM Tansy was just taken to surgery.

9:00 PM Nurse Laurie tells us Tansy is already asleep. Julie and I are moved back into our "suite" in the waiting room.

Day 25

Saturday, July 6, 2002

12:15 AM Dr. Burkett reports the surgery went well. He didn't find any real problems. He drained a bile pocket near the liver, checked the bowel, and put in a chest tube to drain fluid around Tansy's lung. They also removed her appendix.

Jon Hagen and C.S. sat up with us through the surgery- talking.

Pastor Vanman called at 11:40 PM to check on Tansy and us. He called the nurses' station later, too, to check on Tansy.

1:05 AM Tansy was in a lot of pain following surgery. She was extremely alert and aware of her surroundings. Finally, the pain meds took hold, and she settled down. A couple of warm blankets helped to ward off the chills.

The feelings of disappointment and discouragement after learning that I'd be brought back to surgery to have my incision opened back up after three weeks was intense. It was a major incision, over twelve inches, extending from my breastbone to my pubic bone. It was left open to heal from the inside out. Saline moistened gauze was packed into the wound during twice daily bandage changes.

The nurses and my mom were very creative with different techniques to complete my bandage changes without having to use tape to secure them to my body. My skin was so sensitive and fragile that I would get tape burns anytime tape or adhesive was applied to my skin. They fashioned Montgomery straps, looking like a corset, and this is what held the bandages in place while protecting my skin.

Time for all of us to sleep. I pray Tansy can sleep restfully and pain free.

7:10 AM Tansy is awake and wondering about what they did to her in surgery.

7:58 AM Tansy is doing some dreaming, moving her lips, raising her eyebrows, wrinkling her nose and wiggling her toes.

Tansy has a central line, is hooked up to the monitors, has the respirator assisting her, a chest tube machine (the aquarium stocked with tropical fish) is bubbling away- the marvels of modern medicine, it is all very stress producing to see her like this. "Day-by-day" as Dr. Georgen would say.

I'll still feel better when Dr. Wasco gets back.

6:29 PM Julie and Cam are out visiting Grandma Kuchenbecker who just came home from the hospital today with her newly repaired knee.

I went to Clintonville earlier to pick up Cam and to trim vines. The bittersweet is going crazy on the pine trees. Boston ivy needed a haircut on the pergola.

The cats were okay, so was Rex, the betta fish. Geddie stopped by to mow the lawn, but Camden had beat him to it.

Tansy is resting comfortably tonight. Her fever seems to be down. She had a little chicken broth, a few bites of lime Jello, and a couple nibbles of a lemon ice frozen treat. Apple juice continues to go down the best of all.

Theda Star brought in a trauma patient a little while ago. Now I hear it getting ready to leave again.

I'm so happy and relieved to see Tansy feeling better today. Yesterday was so scary and trying on all of us.

7:00 PM Tansy's temp is normal!

7:35 PM Grandpa Sweet is holding Tansy's hand to keep it warm so the O2 sensor stops beeping.

I've battled cold hands ever since my hospital stay following my crash. The oxygen saturation monitor doesn't read as well on a cold finger. Due to this, the monitor would indicate that my O2 levels were below normal by beeping. My grandpa would comfort me by holding my hand in his big, warm hand. Some people are blessed with naturally warm hands. He was one of those people.

Earlier today, Tansy was given some fresh frozen plasma. Now she's getting two units of blood.

Day 26

Sunday, July 7,2002

7:26 AM Camden and I slept at Grandma and Grandpa Sweet's house last night. Julie stayed with Tansy until midnight, working to keep her temperature down.

I called Nurse Laurie at 1:21 AM to check on Tansy and Julie. She told me Tansy's temp was down, and she was resting comfortably (Julie had gone to bed.)

Julie got up at 4:30 AM to take Tansy's temp and then went back to sleep until I walked in at 6:45 AM.

Laurie said Tansy isn't coughing as much as the day of surgery because of the pain. She's guarding herself because of the fresh incision and the chest tube.

We put a pillow on her belly and have her hug it when she needs to cough. It is extremely painful for the poor girl. She was able to get some of the secretions out on her own, and Laurie suctioned out some more. Now she's sleeping again.

Splinting my abdomen with a pillow or folded blanket provided support to my large incision and reduced pain slightly during activities that involved the use of my abdominal muscles like coughing, sneezing or moving. It sat next to me in bed, so I could grab it at a moment's notice anytime I needed it. Doing so also allowed me to cough and breathe deeper to help clear my lungs.

> *Julie went home to help her mom now. Camden bought Tansy a stuffed piglet who says, "You're brave" among other comforting phrases.*
>
> *7:50 PM Tansy has fluid collecting around her right lung now, too. Both Dr. A. and Dr. Burkett are recommending a chest tube on that side. We're waiting for Dr. Burkett to perform the procedure in Tansy's room. This is the third unexpected "procedure" in five days. All of us agree that this is no fun- especially Tansy.*

The trauma didn't end with the crash. It continued in the hospital in ways I never expected. One of the hardest parts was the unknown. The unexpected is part of what makes trauma and hospitals a place of vulnerability and uncertainty. I've always been one who got through life with a carefully planned schedule. My schedule was lost on that highway twenty-six days earlier. Every day since then was completely out of my control, and no matter how hard I fought, I couldn't regain direction of my life.

I'd just had another major abdominal operation where my incision was left gaping open, and I was faced with the placement of yet another chest tube. The setbacks and procedures were getting to be overwhelming, and I didn't know if they'd ever end.

Looking back now, I realize that surviving wasn't just about what my body endured. It was also about facing the unknown. It was about finding emotional strength in moments I didn't think I could handle.

8:01 PM I've sent a record number of thank you notes.

However, the doctor bills are beginning to outnumber the get-well cards in the mailbox.

10:07 PM RT Sharon and Nurse Laurie are getting Tansy ready for the chest tube procedure. Dr. B. has a habit of working late on our daughter.

10:35 PM Chest tube is in place. Dr. Burkett tells us he drained 1 ½ liters of fluid before inserting the tube. There was more fluid surrounding Tansy's right lung than around the left one.

A chest tube is a "thumb-sized" rigid tube that enters the chest cavity between ribs on either side of the torso. The tube is then hooked up to a cannister called a "Pleur-evac," which typically sits on the floor as it needs to be in an upright position, sitting below the level of the patient's trunk.

The fact they removed one and a half liters of fluid is an impressive amount, but I don't specifically recall feeling any sort of relief from this intervention. I attribute that to the array of other injuries and disease processes going on throughout the rest of my body.

I now have mirror image scars on either side of my ribcage from these tubes. Autumn and I later got matching tattoos under our chest tube scars to symbolize what we went through and survived.

10:50 PM Julie goes to bed with a headache.

11:30 PM Nurse Laurie gives me permission to go to bed.

Day 27

Monday, July 8, 2002

6:35 AM I've been up since 6:00 AM. Tansy briefly woke up to tell me she slept okay through the night. Her temp is 99.8 degrees. She's sleeping again.

Laurie said she hurt when they did her chest X-ray at 5:00 AM- the result of the new chest tube along with other things.

Julie's sleeping- I hope that headache went away.

Our heron friend was back on watch duty by the spillway earlier this morning.

1:15 PM Tansy has a high-tech inflatable Hill Rom hospital bed. It is currently positioned like a chair with Tawny in it.

This bed reminded me of a transformer in the way that it converted itself and changed shape. I recall sitting up in bed like this only once. Typically, they'd have me sit in the cardiac chair or at the edge of the bed. It was better for my recovery to have me go through the motions and the work of getting into that position versus having the bed do the work for me.

Dr. Sears said his partner, Dr. M., will probably take care of Tansy's toe problem sometime this week.

3:00 PM Dr. M. shows up to evaluate Tansy's foot (we missed him). He has a foot slipper and pump put on Tansy's foot to reduce swelling.

7:30 PM Brian comes with Lisa N.

9:20 PM Julie and I go to bed early tonight. Tansy gets some zzz's, too. Temp is normal!

12:00 Midnight- Julie gets up to help nurse Laurie turn Tansy. They change dressings and start the bed moving.

Day 28

Tuesday, July 9, 2002

6:00 AM Nurse Laurie tells me to tiptoe out so Tansy can get an extra hour of sleep before the docs start coming. I told her to let Dr. M. know we want to talk with him when he arrives. I might as well lay down for a little longer.

7:12 AM Tansy is still asleep. I'm still waiting for Dr. M. I wrote down some questions to ask him.

1:00 PM Tansy used the Passy Muir tracheostomy and ventilator speaking valve today to talk. Ginger and another PT had her sitting at the bedside for 15 minutes. She seemed to tolerate it well.

This step forward was exhausting but such progress. We were limited by a short leash on the chest tubes, so we settled for sitting at the edge of the bed. Each time I did this, it helped engage muscles, strengthen my core and promote circulation. It was slowly helping me regain strength along with physical, mental and emotional benefits. I felt more in control and less anxious when I was able to successfully complete the therapy session for the day. Ginger was a consistent and encouraging part of this process.

7:05 PM Tansy had a pretty good day. Her temp stayed under control. I don't think her pain was too out of hand.

God, I pray the unexpected twists and turns stop coming.

Sarah's dad and Adam come to visit. Adam is home from Florida to help Sarah's dad go through her things.

Adam is Sarah's brother. She and I traveled to Florida together with her parents to attend his wedding a few years earlier. She loved him so much. He was always the "cool" older brother. She looked forward to the times he was able to come back to Wisconsin to visit and spend time with her.

Tansy's napping. Julie ran out for snacks. Brian and Geddie are coming to visit. Camden is staying at Parry's.

Julie is giving away worry stones with words like trust, peace, love, prayer, etc to anxious relatives in the CCU waiting room.

This explains my mom so well: always worrying about and caring for others. At this point, after four weeks in the hospital with me, she had learned lessons no textbook could ever teach her. Not by choice but by necessity. Grief doesn't need to be fixed. But it does need presence, time and grace.

Those other families that she and my dad met during their time in the CCU became their support in times of need. They spoke, shared stories and traded advice. But my mom's simple worry stone gifts, topped with words of encouragement, didn’t need an explanation.

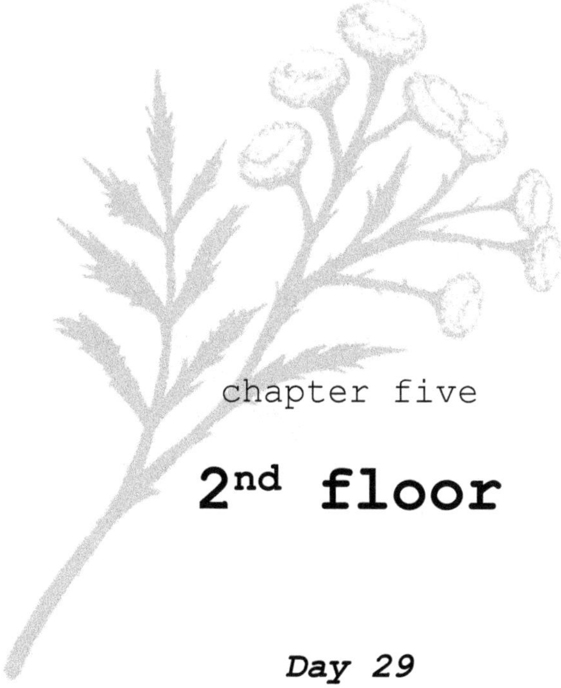

chapter five

2nd floor

Day 29

July 10, 2002

6:32 AM Tawny wants to sleep. I peeked in here a half hour ago. Tansy said, "I'm tired." So, I let her sleep.

Now Dr. Wasco stepped in and is taking out one of her chest tubes. That's a good sign. They had me step out.

7:00 AM Dr. Wasco believes the ERCP was successful in sealing the bile leak. A great sign! Based on today's chest x-ray, they will determine if Tansy can move up to the 2nd floor and out of the CCU (for good, we hope).

Heather G. and her family visited again yesterday. They are such nice people. I just reread the letter she wrote to Tansy; she is such a sweetheart!

11:40 AM Tansy is moving up to 241 sometime between 1:00 and 3:00 PM. Yahoo! Julie is upstairs getting the room decorated for Tansy's arrival.

12:00 Noon The speech therapist watches Tansy eat her first solid food since the accident. She has part of a grilled cheese sandwich and a bite of a pear.

Therapy of any kind was not enjoyable, but it was necessary. Speech therapy was one of my least favorite therapies during this time. Food did not taste good. Everything was flavorless and dry. My sense of smell and taste were off due to breathing through a tube in my neck.

4:00 PM Tansy gets moved back up to room 241.

5:30 PM Tansy is snoozing in her bed on her special air mattress as the CPM machine exercises her left leg.

Julie is taking a nap on her roll-a-way cot in the corner. The left side chest tube is still in place.

Tansy's room has a view of the Oak Street bridge and the new Neenah Public Library from where I'm sitting.

7:10 PM Brian and a host of other friends come up to visit Tawny.

8:40 PM An RT is giving Tansy a breathing treatment as she listens to music.

And we were back on the 2nd floor. I can recall them referring to it as "the step-down unit." It's where patients went when they were still sick, but not sick enough to be in the critical care unit any longer.

My mom decorated my room each time I was transferred to a different unit. She had brought all my photos from home and made several photo collages. These adorned the white walls of my hospital rooms. There were photos of me with my friends, photos of Sarah, sports photos, silly photos, photo booth photos, school photos, many different, memory-provoking pictures.

In addition to the collages, there were big posterboards and banners with messages written from friends and family. There were balloons of varying sizes with different healing phrases on them. There was a large 8"x10" school photo of me from my junior year that my parents had printed on photo paper from their computer at home. This was their way of showing the staff what I used to look like, as I was hard to recognize initially after the crash.

She was able to make my room bright and cheery compared to the standard hospital room. Healthcare workers would frequently comment on the decorations and photos in my room and the effort that went into making it look this way.

Day 30

July 11, 2002

8:13 AM Tansy had a pretty good night. Julie stayed in the room with her. There are frequent interruptions, of course, when the nurses come in.

Dr. Wasco said the chest tube needs to stay in on the left side for another day or two. Her WBCs are down to 22,000. The bile drains look good with little drainage accumulating.

Dr. Sears thinks Tansy's big toe on the right foot is looking infected. He'll have Dr. M. look at it today. He pulled her from eating and drinking thinking the foot surgery may come later today.

Our poor girl has had so much to deal with. We pray this will be the last major obstacle.

9:30 AM Dr. M. came in to look at Tansy's foot. He said he could do the surgery today or wait until Monday. He didn't seem to think her big toe was infected. He didn't think things would demarcate much more.

When he asked Tansy when she'd prefer to have the surgery she said, "sooner rather than later."

He explained to her that she'll have a dressing on her foot for 2-3 weeks along with a fiberglass splint.

After it heals, she will have an orthotic made that will fit inside her shoe. Her balance and walking shouldn't be affected too much by the loss of her toes.

Finding out I'd be losing the toes on my right foot was of such significance to me. Amputation is drastic and can change so much about the way you see yourself.

10:30 AM KC came up and prayed with us.

Dr. Whiteside listened to her lungs. He said the liver injury resulted in a swollen diaphragm which further irritated her lungs. She still has some pockets of fluid around her right lung which hopefully will be absorbed by her body. The left side is still draining through the chest tube which will remain in place.

I've been walking through the halls for the past hour and 15 minutes while the nurse did a bath, dressing change, linens, etc. The worry stones are getting their share of rubbing today, believe me.

Julie went to Clintonville about two hours ago to stop by the vet, bring Cam back, get mail and money.

Tansy is napping.

12:27 PM Brian just called. He is going to stop in for a visit before work. He sure has been good to Tansy since her accident happened. He calls every day and visits very frequently. Brian is a good boy (friend) for our girl.

Did you know I ended up marrying this guy!?! We've been through a lot together. Most 17-year-old boys wouldn't have stuck around during this type of life-changing, intense trauma. Brian not only stuck around but was in touch with my parents daily and made the hour-long trip to Neenah to visit me several times a week.

Years later, I stood across from that same man, promising forever to the one who had already proven what "in sickness and in health" really means. Now that we're married, he's a hard-working, dinner-making mechanic who can fix or build anything I ask, all while teaching our kids how to love and respect the outdoors through camping, fishing and hunting.

3:58 PM Camden is here now. We went to Taco Bell for some soft-shell tacos.

Now Tansy is having OT with a therapist. They were discussing orchids, painting watercolors, drawing, and reading- ways to pass the time.

5:15 PM They finally wheeled Tansy down to surgery to have the toes on her right foot amputated. I feel so sorry for her.

6:45 PM Dr. M. meets with Julie, Pastor Vanman (he shows up at all the right times), and me to tell us Tansy's foot surgery went well. He sat down and talked to us like he had as much time as we needed.

9:08 PM Tansy is resting more comfortably back in room 241. She was in lots of pain when we met her in the hallway and wheeled her back up here. Despite all the morphine and other drugs given in the OR, Tansy is still aware of what's going on in here; even when she appears to be sleeping.

After being on pain meds and controlled substances continuously for thirty days, it took more medication for me to get the intended pain relief after major surgeries. Having a third of my right foot amputated resulted in acute pain from cutting through skin, muscle and bone, but it also resulted in pain to the missing limb. My brain hadn't yet comprehended that my toes were gone, so the perception of pain continued in the missing limb for some time.

Day 31

July 12, 2002

6:50 AM Tansy had a good night in between being woken up periodically. Julie slept next to her on the cot.

3:00 PM Can you tell it's been a rather uneventful day? That's a good thing. We want lots more of these. That means there is rest and healing going on.

Both Tansy and Julie are napping. I was sitting out in the garden on a perfect summer afternoon.

Tansy had some watermelon, one bite of mac and cheese, and one noodle from her chicken noodle soup. She's been drinking lots of water, apple juice and some OJ too.

7:15 PM Dr. V. came in to talk to us about the rehab unit. Patients in Tansy's condition typically spend 2-4 weeks up there.

He also told Tansy about a drug that soothes the nerves affecting phantom pain (Neurontin).

Phantom pain is a painful perception relating to a limb that is no longer physically a part of the body. This perception for me was very present initially and slowly lessened as time passed and healing occurred. I don't have phantom pain any longer. I do, however, have nerve pain, or residual limb pain. It feels like a sharp, electric-like shock at the end of my foot. I get it mostly when I'm driving home after working all day.

I've found ways to cope with this over the years: gently massaging my limb, changing position, walking on it or some other form of distraction. It doesn't last forever. I can get through anything that only lasts for a few moments.

Dr. Georgen told Tansy she's over the worst part of the recovery. Now she needs to bulk up and eat and build up her strength so she can get home. It looks as though she'll move up to 6th floor by next week.

Hearing this was encouraging, but I didn't feel anywhere near ready to move on to the last step of this hospital journey. Could I do it?

Moving to the 6th floor rehabilitation unit brought with it the requirement to complete intensive physical and occupational therapy on a regular basis. Sometimes I was so emotional, exhausted and defeated that I just didn't feel like participating in hours of therapy. I knew it was important, but so was my mental health and rest. I knew I needed to find a balance.

Day 32

Saturday, July 13, 2002

8:00 AM Dr. Georgen will be pulling the left side chest tube sometime today, we hope. Tansy doesn't have much of an appetite. She ate a few grapes, a bite of banana, a little bit of Rice Krispies cereal, and some apple juice (her mainstay).

She says she loves the taste of Jevity the best.

This was another one of my dad's jokes, as I'm certain I didn't like the taste of any of it. Whether he's referring to my tube feeding or an oral nutritional supplement in this case, none of it was palatable. Apple juice, however, was, and always has been, my favorite beverage.

> *9:00 AM Dr. Georgen pulls Tansy's chest tube, her two Jackson-Pratt drains, and debrides her abdominal incision.*
>
> *She has plans to get in a chair this PM and wheel around.*

Removing the last chest tube and various drains meant moving and breathing was going to be easier and less uncomfortable for me. A JP drain is a surgical suction drain that draws fluid from a wound after a surgical procedure. The bulb connected to an external tube that was several inches long, with approximately 6-8 inches of it inserted into my abdomen through a tiny surgical incision. It was held in place by a stitch. Both drains were in different areas of my abdomen to help remove excess fluid that could complicate healing or cause infection. They were removed when the output from these drains was below a certain level. At that point, they had done their job and were no longer needed.

The process of removing the drains meant cutting a stitch that held them in place and pulling the tube out. I could feel the two JP drain tubes moving through my insides as they were being pulled out of my belly. I recall the large diameter of the chest tube being pulled from between my ribs. It hurt, but once they were out, the discomfort was gone.

I can still recall the times my abdominal incision was debrided. Debridement is the process of removing dead or unhealthy tissue from a wound with a scalpel. This sounds scary and intimidating, but the dead tissue didn't have any sensation, so although it was done without anesthetic, it was not painful.

The day Dr. Georgen came in to tell me three of my tubes could come out felt like progress. But then reality set in. I was still connected to so many things keeping me alive. A tracheostomy tube for breathing, a feeding tube in my stomach, a catheter in my bladder and a couple IVs delivering medications and fluids.

> *12:00 Noon I went to McDonald's to get Tansy some chicken nuggets. She tried one and spit it out. It was too dry. Nothing tastes very good with that trach in place.*

One of my favorite foods was chicken nuggets from McDonalds. Unfortunately, nothing tasted good enough to eat. Except apple juice.

A happy nugget-related memory of Sarah was when the two of us accompanied my mom to Neenah to stay at my grandparents' house for my birthday weekend each November. We would stop at McDonald's on the way out of town and get chicken nugget meals for dinner. I preferred the dark meat, or "wet" nuggets and she preferred the white meat, or "dry" nuggets. So, we traded nuggets accordingly.

4:03 PM Julie finally went to Kuchen-becker's to take a shower.

The nurses have done a good job of letting Tansy (and us) rest this PM. That seems to be the first and foremost thing our girl needs. But she also needs to get out of bed. I hope we can accomplish that tonight.

It's another beautiful, warm summer day. We'll appreciate each one of these more than ever once we get out of here and back into the swing of living more normally.

Camden has a great weekend to be at Kelsey's cottage.

Day 33

Sunday, July 14, 2002

7:19 AM Julie reported to me that Tansy had kind of a rough night after I left. When the nurse tried to irrigate her drain site, Tansy just about went through the roof. Julie asked the nurse to get Dr. Georgen. Luckily, he was able to come up right away.

He stuck a Q-Tip in there and decided to order a CT scan to check things out. That will be done some time today.

Then Tawny threw up. Julie was frazzled, who wouldn't be. This isn't any fun.

5:00 PM Tansy went down for a CT scan around noon to check on the drain site area. Dr. Georgen hasn't been back up because of all the trauma cases that have come in this PM.

A nurse changed Tansy's foot dressing. It was the first time all of us saw Tansy's foot without toes. It was sad for Tansy, but she will deal with it.

The first time I saw my foot after the amputation, my heart sank. I knew the surgeon had removed my toes days before, and I had been told several times it would happen, but nothing could have prepared me for that moment when I looked down and saw it for myself.

The nurse carefully removed the layers of my bulky bandage as my parents and I anxiously watched on. Then she finally removed that last layer of gauze, exposing my new foot. Where my toes had been, there was only emptiness, and at that moment, I felt the weight of everything I had lost.

A psychologist met with her for the first time around 1:30 PM.

Perhaps the timing of meeting with a psychologist for the first time and seeing my newly amputated foot for the first time wasn't coincidental. In general, I was an emotional wreck. The last thing I wanted to do was be forced to talk to a shrink. I certainly didn't request this. I recall that he asked me questions about why I was feeling sad about losing my ability to wear sandals.

He didn't understand my 17-year-old mind, and I didn't feel I made progress from the few discussions we had together.

Julie has been working Tansy's arms and legs, as has a weekend PT. I played a rousing game of balloon ping pong to work on range of motion of her arms.

8:00 PM After talking to Camden on the phone, I decided to go pick him up from Parry's.

9:00 PM We get home and spend the night with Sonny, Sassy and Naughty.

I called Julie and found out Dr. Georgen stopped in and gave the results of Tansy's CT scan. She needs to have fluid pockets drained from around her right lung and her liver.

Day 34

Monday, July 15, 2002

6:00 AM I cut the grass, trimmed and weeded, filled the pond, clipped a few bushes, did three loads of wash, and vacuumed the house.

I dropped Cam off at Parry's, cashed my check, and got back here by 1:30 PM.

Tansy was still having the fluid draining procedure done by Dr. M. There is some thick pus-like junk near her liver, and a drain was put in. It was also cultured, as it was two days ago.

3:06 PM Tansy just got her trach out (it was falling out following her procedure.) Yipee-progress. Now nurse Nancy is removing Tansy's central line. A new IV was placed in her left wrist.

Having my tracheostomy tube removed was a big milestone. It came out easier than I expected it to. It slid right out. A piece of gauze and paper tape temporarily sealed the hole in my neck. I was able to talk without the speaking valve. However, I did have to press my finger over the tape to make an airtight seal to speak until it healed over.

For weeks it had been my lifeline. When it finally came out I felt apprehensive. But I also felt free. Free to breathe, to talk and to move forward. It was proof of progress, a sign that I was getting stronger and closer to recovery.

3:45 PM Another therapy dog stopped in for a visit. This was a very nice golden retriever named Abbie. We wanted to take her home with us. Tansy is on the therapy dog visiting list. Several have stopped by. They are great!!!

Hospital days were tough and dark, but visits from therapy dogs were a temporary ray of light. The most healing moments came when these dogs would stop by just to greet me. If they were small, they'd hop on my bed to snuggle. The bigger ones stayed on the ground but came right up to me, so I could pet them. They were all so well-behaved and friendly. We had golden retrievers growing up, so they were always our favorite four-legged hospital visitors.

Day 35

Tuesday, July 16, 2002

6:42 AM I just arrived at the hospital after a good night's sleep. Tawny is having her vital signs checked. Julie is still in bed but awake. Another day.

1:00 PM We washed Tansy's hair. Julie put it in Pippi Longstocking French braids.

Having my hair washed felt amazing. The nurse used an inflatable hair basin under my head while I was flat in bed. In a basin of warm water, she and my mom washed my hair with shampoo and conditioner. I enjoyed a grape flavored popsicle during this experience. Afterwards, my mom brushed my hair and French braided it in pigtails. She frequently had it in this style to keep the wound on the back of my head free of hair to help it to heal.

Tansy checked her email and played solitaire on the laptop computer that Jon Hagen arranged for her to use.

I still have handwritten instructions from Jon, in his signature handwriting, on how to operate the laptop.

Technology has changed so much in the last twenty-three years. Back then, we didn't carry the internet in our pockets or purses. We had a bulky desktop computer with dialup internet. No one could use the land line while someone was "surfing the web."

Back in the hospital, it was a nice break to have the option to use the laptop for a bit. I sat in bed with the computer over my lap on the bedside table. Social media didn't exist yet. There was no Facebook or Instagram to scroll through aimlessly.

The main method of communication as a 17-year-old in 2002 was calling someone's house on a landline, riding a bike over to a friend's house or passing a folded-up note to someone as you passed them in the hall at school. I certainly didn't have a fan club of unread emails to check.

Tansy is moving around more easily in bed. Her pain seems better today. She must get off the Morphine PCA pump before she gets to 6th floor.

She's supposed to get up and into a wheelchair at 2:00 PM. I hope that goes well and we get to move to rehab, soon!

4:07 PM Tansy was transferred from a sitting position into a regular wheelchair at 2:30 PM. We went to 6th floor, down to CCU, and around the 1st floor by the garden. It was the first time out of her room in a chair in about two weeks. That is more positive progress.

This was also the first time I was in a standard wheelchair and not the cardiac chair. I had to support myself with my core muscles as I sat upright, my head had to remain clear, and my arms and legs were on their corresponding rests. It was tiring, but I was doing it.

Lots of visitors tonight: Sarah and Ryan, Brian, Geddie and Alicia, Patty and Lindsay.

6:30 PM Dr. P. of rehab checks Tansy over and gives her the okay to move into room 677.

Dr. Burkett holds Tansy's hand and tells the miracle girl she's ready to move upstairs. Now just Dr. M. must give his okay.

An infectious disease doctor tells us the thick yellow substance by Tansy's liver is yeast, a result of extended antibiotic treatment. He'll cut back on one of those and treat the yeast with an anti-fungal medication. He gives us the thumbs up sign. We are extremely happy and relieved.

After several weeks, I had finally reached the last step of my hospital journey: rehab. I knew the hardest work was still to come. This was where I would learn to do the everyday things I once took for granted: standing, moving and caring for myself.

Getting to rehab wasn't just another transfer to a different hospital unit, it was a milestone. It meant I had survived the worst, and now I had the opportunity to remake myself.

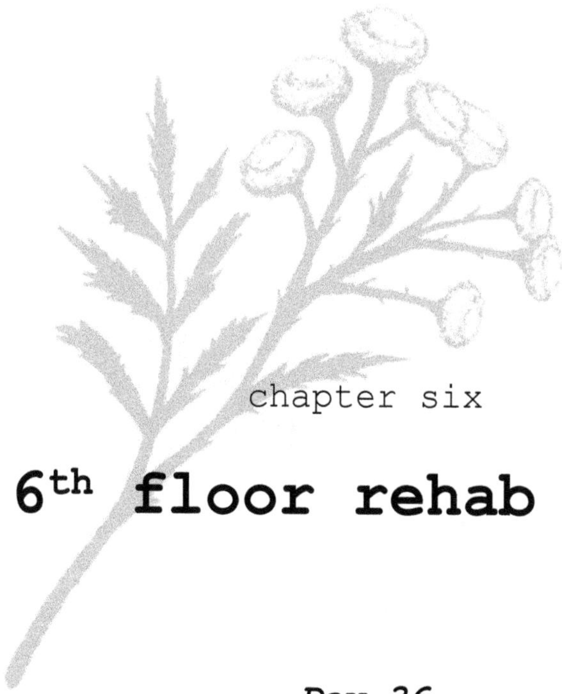

chapter six

6th floor rehab unit

Day 36

Wednesday, July 17, 2002

7:39 AM Julie left to take a shower.

Dr. M. with orthopedics just peeked in to ask how Tansy is doing. Swelling in her thighs is a sign of healing. Popping during exercises with PT is tendons rubbing over screw heads. If it persists, screws can be surgically removed after bones have healed.

Tansy's still sleeping from a 4:00 AM dose of Ativan given to help her relax.

Someone is changing the suction canister that is drawing Tansy's stomach contents out. She still is having trouble tolerating her G-tube being clamped for extended periods of time. She becomes nauseated after a while. She also has a J-tube.

I received nutrition in the form of a tube feeding through a tube in my stomach for several weeks. It was an orange-colored substance, and I swear I was able to taste it. This was likely my brain playing tricks on me as I was desperate to eat something that tasted good again.

10:30 AM Tansy was crying and in lots of pain when Ginger and Tammy came in to do therapy at 8:00 AM. They were going to get her into a chair at 9:00 AM instead, but that didn't work either. They'll be back this afternoon.

Julie decided to go to Clintonville to spend time with Camden.

If Tansy is having a rough day I wonder if they'll just keep her here instead of going up to 6th floor.

1:30 PM Tansy moved up to the penthouse suite 677. Ginger transferred her to a wheelchair for the event. Tansy wasn't feeling too well when she arrived.

3:52 PM I got all of Tansy's things moved up here while she rested. When Julie gets here, we can decide if we want to put everything up or not. This room is very bright with the southern and western exposure.

Pat T. popped her head in to say hello to Tansy.

5:00 PM Julie is back with Rex (Tansy's betta fish).

Rex was the betta fish Brian got me prior to my crash. He picked him out and named him. He was a special gift for me at the time. I cherished everything that Brian got for me during our young years together. It was always something so meaningful to me.

I love that my mom brought my pet to the hospital to keep me company while I was in rehab. I previously had a photo of him taped on my hospital wall, as he wasn't allowed in the CCU and perhaps not the 2nd floor either.

Eagle III, a competing air medical rescue service from Brown County, landed here with a patient.

Day 37

Thursday, July 18, 2002

7:28 AM Julie and Tansy continue to sleep as I sit outside the room in the lounge with a view. The night nurse told me Tansy had a good sleep thanks in part to Ativan.

I wonder what today will bring. I hope for less pain, an appetite, and more ease of movement. Less stress and fear would be welcomed also.

1:00 PM The case manager just told us the rehab team met to discuss Tansy's case. Once she eats, bulks up, and learns to transfer from a wheelchair to bed, to car, to toilet- she can go home in two to three weeks- maybe sooner.

She could work on rehab as an outpatient and continue to visit her doctors. Outpatient rehab could be done closer to home- perhaps right in Clintonville.

Two to three weeks!?! I was determined to get home sooner than that. I knew what I had to do, and I was going to work hard and make it happen. At that moment, I never realized it would take me only six days.

5:30 PM Lots of friends came to visit. Uncle Randy and I went out to eat using one of many food gift certificates received from staff at school.

Prior to the crash, one of our big summer plans were for Sarah S., Sarah D., Becca, Alicia and I to take a trip to Rock Island in Door County. This trip did not end up happening as originally planned, but Sarah D., Becca and Alicia were still able to go together. They brought along a blown-up white balloon with a sharpie face drawn on it to symbolize me on their trip. They took several photos, then came to visit me afterwards while I was in rehab to fill me in and tell me all about it.

Day 38

Friday, July 19, 2002

8:43 AM Tansy and Julie had lots of interruptions during the night. An old friend of Tansy's showed up at 9:15 PM to visit. Julie let him stay for about 5 minutes.

Nurses had trouble with the feeding IV beeping, three shots were given in Tansy's butt (pneumonia, flu and meningitis).

6:43 PM I picked up Camden and Kelsey at about 1:15 PM. We stopped at a car dealership in Appleton and test drove a BMW (to benefit breast cancer research and because it was fun.)

When we got back, we met Autumn Henry of Shiocton. She was in a car accident in March that left her paralyzed from the waist down. She came up to meet Tansy and us. What a sweet, pretty, and inspirational girl. Amy Johnson has been mentoring her. Both arranged to meet N.S. and her parents. She'll be going to Froedtert to rehab just as Amy did.

Tansy practiced car transfers in the OT/PT gym this PM. Ginger let Camden and Kelsey use a wheelchair so they could join us as we went for a walk with Tansy.

Amy Johnson visited with Tansy and me while Julie took Kelsey and Camden out to dinner.

That was the first time I met Autumn after previously hearing my parents talk about her. I have a photo of us together from that moment. She looked gorgeous, and I was in rough shape, but it was the first of many photos of us together. I recently asked Autumn what stood out to her from our first time meeting each other. She told me, "I remember crying the whole way home because my heart felt your broken heart's heaviness."

Meeting Autumn was like finding someone who could understand a language that few others spoke. We both carried the weight of trauma. Our scars didn't always show but shaped how we moved through life. We found comfort in sharing those exposed and unhealed pieces of ourselves. Our similarities didn't just connect us; they built the foundation for a friendship that has lasted ever since.

The details of our experiences were different, but some of our emotions were the same: loss, fear, pain and the fight to keep moving forward. In each other, we found someone who didn't need long explanations or justification. We understood without words.

We became bonded by trauma. Not in a way we ever would have chosen, but in a way that has given us a rare kind of friendship. One that runs deeper and reminds us that we are not alone in the hard parts of life.

Day 39

Saturday, July 20, 2002

12:35 PM We took Tansy down to the main entrance with PT to practice a wheelchair/car transfer to our Pontiac Vibe. With the seat back and reclined the transfer went well.

Tansy has kind of a touchy stomach yet, however. She vomited in bed after we got her back up to the room.

Dr. M. with pulmonology removed the tape covering the opening where her trach had been. That was upsetting to her. It must heal the rest of the way uncovered. Her voice sounds hoarse, and she didn't like seeing the hole in her throat. It will be completely closed in a few days.

When my trach tube was initially removed, tape covered the remaining circular opening. When the doctor took the tape off, it hurt my overly sensitive skin. I preferred the tape covering it as it felt protected. Now with the tape removed, it felt exposed, naked and vulnerable. I couldn't speak unless I covered the hole with my finger. I could hear the air escaping through the hole, and it would whistle at times.

Tansy wants to get out of the hospital ASAP. I echo those sentiments completely.

Dennis and Kay just arrived for a visit. They went with Julie downstairs to get lunch before the cafeteria closes.

7:35 PM Julie went home to Kuchenbecker's to take a little break from the hospital.

Bonnie and Jay came to get Camden and Kelsey.

9:00 PM The three of us are back together in penthouse suite 677.

My parents referred to it as the "penthouse" because it was on the 6th floor of the hospital which was also the top. It was the very end room, on the corner with two windows overlooking the helipad and the Fox River. It's now referred to as "the room with a view" by my dad and me.

Day 40

Sunday, July 21, 2002

6:53 AM Very dark clouds are moving across the sky creating an ominous start to the day.

The girls are still snoozing, although Tansy appears to be awake.

I'm watching the wind make changing patterns on the harbor water. The sailboats indicate a north wind.

The helicopter is being wheeled into the hanger to protect it from the approaching storms.

I'm waiting for Dr. Wasco to make his rounds.

10:30 AM Tansy gets her first ride in a car in 40 days. We drove for a quick trip to see Grandma Kuchenbecker who came out using her walker to say hi to Tansy in the Pontiac Vibe. It's a big day.

We decide not to stop anywhere else because Tansy's stomach feels upset.

I recall this first car ride. It was nerve-wracking being in a vehicle again after the last time ended the way it did. I'm sure my parents were very aware that I'd feel this way, so they kept the drive short and stuck to city roads, as I got motion sick easily.

But taking that first ride also became one of the biggest triumphs in my recovery. Each mile reminded me that I was stronger than my fear, that I could face the very thing that had changed my life forever.

12:00 Noon Now she's back in bed resting after receiving a pain pill. The morphine was discontinued yesterday. The narcotic patch is in place on Tansy's left deltoid. A PT is exercising her legs.

Julie is running errands. Camden is at Kelsey's. It is very hot and muggy for Neenah's annual "Art in the Park" event.

1:35 PM Rod and Nancy stopped by for a visit. Tansy is feeling a little nauseated. She's wide awake and listening to the story of her stay in the hospital. So far, we've gotten to day 9 of the 40-day saga.

This was the first time I heard the story, written from my dad's perspective, of what happened on Wednesday, June 12, 2002, at 4:18 PM through the first several days of my hospital stay. It was surreal, like listening to someone else's story, only it was mine. I learned how close I had come to not making it. Hearing it all was overwhelming, but it also gave me perspective. It reminded me not only of the pain I had endured but of the strength, love and miracles that carried me through.

8:49 PM The night heron is watching from the fence as he has been most of the day. I'm on watch, too. Julie finally agreed to give herself a break and is sleeping at Morris and Jean's house.

Dark storm clouds are drifting in from the northwest. I'm hoping for a display of nature's fireworks over beautiful downtown Neenah.

Tansy was awake and talking more than ever today. The end of the morphine is helping that, I think.

Nurse Jackie gave her something to settle her stomach. The tube feeding has been discontinued so Tansy needs to drink to keep from getting dehydrated.

Once her stomach settles down and gets used to eating again, she'll be headed home.

It was 99 degrees outside at 5:10 PM when Julie and I went to eat dinner.

Day 41

July, 22, 2002

9:27 AM Tansy is getting a new IV site put in. The other one isn't working anymore. We were bunkies last night. She had a good night with only minor interruptions.

Dr. Wasco came and took out Tansy's G and J feeding tubes. Now she's really got to eat and drink on her own.

8:03 PM Tansy has been awake since 2:30 PM when she had OT and PT. Less medication means a more alert Tansy.

She just had a jar of Gerber baby food peaches- whatever it takes to get her stomach going.

When my feeding tube was removed in the hospital, it was another big step forward. But it came with a new challenge. My appetite was almost nonexistent. Food didn't sound good, and eating felt like a chore. It felt more like a mountain I had no energy to climb.

Still, I knew I had to start nourishing my body to keep healing. If I wanted my massive, open abdominal wound to heal, I needed to eat. If I wanted to gain back the tremendous amount of weight I had lost, I needed to eat. If I wanted the fresh incision on my right foot to heal, I needed to eat. Strength wasn't going to come without work, and I needed sustenance and protein to build myself back up.

Taking pills in applesauce isn't much better than the ice cream method.

We're watching a video- "A Walk in the Clouds"- nothing too special.

Julie went home and bought a double bed for Tansy at Mitchell's. It's already set up. Several friends are helping Julie repaint Tansy's room so it will be fresh and inviting when we arrive home on a weekend pass this Friday.

The sun is setting over the industrial Fox River and its paper mills, bridges and railroad trestles.

My mom and seventeen of my friends had a painting party at my house. They painted my bedroom walls and ceiling blue and added pink swirls. Everyone put their handprint on the ceiling along with their initials. Matt decided to do a footprint instead. (I would loved to have witnessed this.) Brian somehow managed to kiss the ceiling. And my mom wrote "MOM" under her handprint in all capital letters.

In the end, there were roughly twenty bright pink handprints with corresponding initials, one set of lips and a random footprint on my ceiling. I loved every single one of them. Once I was home, I was eventually able to lie in my bed, look up at my ceiling and pick out who each set of prints and initials belonged to. These prints reminded me of the love and support I had from so many of my friends.

I have several photos from this specific event, since I couldn't be there in person. Josh painted his entire face blue, and Matt hung upside down from the beam in the vaulted living room. I'm certain I recall hearing that a few of the guys took a dip in the pond behind our house as well.

12:00 Midnight- A shooting star streaked across the northwest sky as I lay sleepless on the cot- a good omen.

Day 42

Tuesday, July 23, 2002

6:19 AM Tansy slept soundly the whole night except around 3:00 AM when she had to use the bedpan. I repositioned her a couple times, and she turned herself the other times.

It's a beautiful morning. We're hoping for a great day.

8:05 AM Tansy "drank" some of her baby food peaches, had a couple bites of an English muffin, a few bites of melon, some apple and grape juice. Now she's taking another snooze.

Dr. Wasco said she can take a shower today. Tammy showed her the shower setup yesterday. She'll be ready to do that after Dr. M. gives his okay.

9:21 AM Tansy's first hospital bill for June 12- July 17 is $234,000. Rehab bills separately from July 17-July 23 are over $10,000.

11:15 AM OT Tammy is giving Tansy her first shower in 42 days.

Earlier, Ann Y. and Jon Hagen stopped in for a visit.

The S. Family brought Tansy a going away gift. Their daughter is being transferred to the spinal cord rehab center at Froedtert Hospital in Milwaukee.

12:25 PM Tansy enjoyed her shower.

4:00 PM Julie was so excited about painting Tansy's room with 17 of our girl's friends that she got us a pass to go home today. Jon Hagen saw us to the door.

6:30 PM We're eating Subway sandwiches at home; we're a family again!

Tansy is in the recliner next to the fireplace bending her knees. Brian and Geddie are over. Camden is popping wheelies in Tansy's chair.

I made it home! For a test run at least, to see how I do outside the safety net of doctors, nurses and constant monitoring.

Another photo memory here. We were in the living room; I was sitting in the maroon recliner next to the fireplace with a soft, chenille, cream-colored blanket on my lap. Brian was sitting next to me holding my hand. I was wearing new pink pajamas that my mom bought for me since none of my old clothes fit properly. On the fireplace next to me, was a glass of apple juice, a pink container of scented body butter and the cordless house phone. All the necessities. We were engaged in a conversation with our other friends who had stopped by.

Sitting there with my friends and family, visiting and laughing in the comfort of our living room was such a nice change compared to the hospital setting that we had all grown accustomed to.

I was so excited to finally sleep in my own bed with my soft flannel sheets. Home felt familiar, yet everything about me had changed. That night reminded me how far I'd come, but also how much adjusting still lay ahead.

chapter seven

discharged

Day 43

Wednesday, July 24, 2002

12:24 PM We're back at the hospital but none of us want to be here anymore. If everything is okay, we may be blowing this pop stand for good later. Dr. P. is checking into this possibility.

3:00 PM Tawny gets fitted for a different wheelchair. Tansy had more physical therapy with Ginger. She stands supporting herself on the parallel bars. Julie gets a migraine and lies down in room 673.

I've got several photos of me and Ginger working together in the gym. Standing at the parallel bars was difficult, but I'd come a long way from the first time I stood after the crash. She put a gait belt around my waist, but I did a lot of the work with my arms to support myself on the bars.

I've also got a photo of us practicing the wheelchair/car transfers in the physical therapy gym. There was part of an old vehicle with front seats for patients to practice getting in and out of. In the photo, my mom was leaning on the hood of the brown vehicle, watching the progress through the windshield. Ginger was assisting me in my wheelchair as I got positioned properly next to the passenger seat of the vehicle with the door open.

4:00 PM Tansy is officially discharged with a huge list of meds. The car is crammed to the gills with 6 weeks of accumulated junk and the wheelchair.

A nurse drops Rex on the pavement. We rescue him and put him and his water in a plastic waste basket.

Julie is so sick she stays overnight at her parents' house.

After forty-three days in the hospital, I was finally discharged to go home. When the time came, things didn't go quite how I pictured.

My mom had a migraine so severe that she had to stay in Neenah. That meant my dad and I went home together to Clintonville for the very first night outside the safety of the hospital.

I was worried about him having to do the "nurse" things that my mom would typically do. I know he was worried about it too. He later told me he was terrified of doing it himself.

My mom was incredibly tough and resilient. She wouldn't have stayed in Neenah if she didn't have to.

For so long, the hospital had been my security blanket, even with all the pain and challenges, I was never far from help.

6:00 PM Tansy and I drive home. I called the neighbor kid to help me get her up the ping pong table ramp. Then I go to Erickson's to get her meds and dressings.

Reading this made me smile. We had two or three steps in the garage to get into the house. We had a thick heavy-duty ping pong table that my parents had decided to use to get my wheelchair into the house for the first day. The next day, a carpenter came over and built a wooden ramp in the garage, so I could wheel in and out of the house.

7:00 PM Back at home. A retired nurse and neighbor administer Tansy's Lovenox injection. I muddled through the rest. Visitors come.

9:20 PM Visitors asked to leave. I changed Tansy's dressing and helped her in the bathroom. Bed time at last.

This was the first night at home after a long unexpected six-week journey. This is the end of the forty-three-day journal my dad kept about my car crash and hospital stay. The last quarter of his journal is titled, “Home Chapter.” He continued to label them by days, even though we were out of the hospital, but the saga and healing was far from over.

chapter eight

home: a new normal

My mom arrived home from Neenah early the next morning. Both my dad and I were relieved and happy to have her there with us. It was good to be home and get into the grove of our new normal. This included frequent doctor's visits, several medications, daily bandage changes, physical therapy multiple times a week, a lot of rest, visits from friends and family and eating to try to gain back some weight.

When I first got home, I was unable to walk and needed a fair amount of help with transfers and moving from one place to the next. I'm not sure who came up with the idea, but I used a doorbell as a method of signaling for help when I needed it. The button itself was on the shelf on my bed for me to push when I needed assistance. The chime was in the living room, so when it rang, it could be heard from the main areas of the house. We were so used to having a call light in the hospital for this purpose.

Sometimes the hardest steps we'll ever take are the ones most people take for granted. After the crash, and forty-three days in the hospital, I had to relearn how to walk. What once felt automatic suddenly became a challenge. Every step was painful and uncertain.

A little over a week after being home from the hospital, I started walking with a walker. Less than ten days later, I was walking without assistance and climbing stairs.

A month after being home, my mom wrote me the following letter, typed in her signature all caps and printed on colored paper with pink and yellow tulips around the perimeter:

8-20-02

DEAR TANSY,

I AM SORRY THAT YOU HAVE LOST YOUR BEST FRIEND, SARAH. HOLD ON TO THE HAPPY MEMORIES AND ALWAYS KEEP HER IN YOUR HEART. I WILL BE RIGHT HERE FOR YOU ALWAYS... TO LAUGH WITH, CRY AND HOLD YOU WHEN YOU'RE SAD.

I LOVE YOU, TAWNY.

LOVE,

MOM

My new normal meant adjusting to a life and a body that had been altered in an instant. Simple things took more time, patience and courage than I could've imagined.

Coming home from the hospital after forty-three days was supposed to feel like the finish line, but really, it was just the start of another chapter. On day 81, I went to an evening football game with friends in Clintonville. It didn't end well for me.

Day 81

Saturday, August 31, 2002

Tansy came home at 10:30 PM feeling dizzy, weak and chilled. Julie got her ready for bed. Then later in the night she took her temperature- 102.8 degrees Fahrenheit.

This morning it's 100 degrees. We called Dr. Wasco's office, spoke with the on-call surgeon and explained the situation. He asked if the drain site had closed off (it had). He suggested hot compresses and expressing it.

Tansy threw up when Julie tried to give her some baby peaches.

I don't like this. Please, God, don't let this start up again.

1:00 PM Dr. B. has us come to the ER for blood work and a CT scan. Scan looks better, WBCs up to 18,000. Tansy has chills and fever. Stent from ERCP is suspect. Takes urine culture to check for bladder infection.

Tansy gets admitted to Children's Hospital of Wisconsin- Fox Valley on the Theda Clark Medical Center campus.

Just over eighty days since the crash (and thirty-eight days after being home from my forty-three-day hospital stay), I was readmitted to the hospital with complications.

I felt like I was reliving it all over again. The major difference was I knew exactly what was going on this time around. I was aware of the happenings in the emergency room, the tests, the IV start, the blood draws and I was awake while they performed a CT scan of my abdomen. The major similarity? My parents were there too, supporting me the whole time.

Day 82

Sunday, September 1, 2002

Julie stayed overnight with Tansy. Noisy vent kept them both awake in room 404 until Julie complained and got moved to 428/429- the isolation room.

I haven't been a great sleeper since the car crash. I specifically recall having a difficult time sleeping with the extra noise during that admission.

This morning, while I was at Bethany Free Church, giving my Tansy testimonial, the doctor tried to remove the stent. He did it under heavy sedation in Tansy's hospital room. He couldn't get it out. Tansy felt much of what he was doing and was very uncomfortable. I guess they'll have to put her out in the OR to remove the stent.

They are going to observe her for 24 hours then send her home. She has a bladder infection. We'd like the stent out before she goes home. Otherwise, we're going to have to do this all over again.

I ended up having a repeat ERCP to remove the stent as an outpatient. It was successful.

Julie is napping. Brian and Tansy are watching a movie. Grandma and Grandpa Sweet stopped up, as did Jon and Pam Hagen.

Last night a group of eight friends came by. Today, Becca, Lindsay, Annika and Alicia stopped in, too. Tansy sure has some loyal, close friends. She's lucky.

8:08 PM Julie went to sleep at home in Clintonville. I'm staying with Tansy in isolation room 429.

Jon and Pam Hagen stopped by to visit Tansy this PM. Julie gave Pam an antique milk carton. I gave Jon several of my articles to read.

Tansy feels better tonight. It appears we'll be going home tomorrow.

Day 83

Monday, September 2, 2002

7:00 AM "What are you doing back here?" I heard that from the cafeteria woman while I was eating breakfast.

Last night I took Tansy down to CCU to show her photo album to the nurses. Both Laurie and Lori were there and a couple of the telemetry girls. They seemed very glad to see us and instantly looked at the pictures.

I get very strong feelings when I pass through that waiting room and when I see patients in those rooms. That place is full of intense memories.

Tomorrow school starts. I guess it was fitting that we should end this summer back in the hospital. Fitting but not preferred.

This concludes the entries I've shared from my dad's journal during one of the most difficult times in my entire life. His "Home Chapter" entries continue for several more weeks, but the intense and acute phase was mostly over. I'm so thankful he kept such a detailed account during that time. It offered me a unique perspective that I wouldn't have otherwise had. It showed me the strength, love and voice that my parents had while I was working to regain mine.

Like my dad, I still get very strong feelings being back at Theda Clark to this day. I like to stop out in the garden, which is completely enclosed by the building with a winding path, flowers, trees and benches. I have flashbacks from going out there during my original hospital stay. I could walk past the old waiting room of the CCU or the elevator bank, and it would bring back vivid memories of my time there.

I can still picture my mom taking me to the crash site for the first time, driving down the highway together and pulling off to the side of the road when we reached our destination. For some reason, I envisioned the site of the crash being at the old intersection where the state highway met highway 29 just outside of Green Bay. I didn't realize that we'd only made it six minutes out of Clintonville.

I saw the cross with pink flowers and the memorial set up for Sarah on the side of the road. There was a photo of us from a dance we had previously attended together. There was a softball with signatures on it. There were several flowers, a stuffed animal and a letter that someone had written to her.

I could feel the lump in my throat rise as I looked over the meticulously placed items symbolizing seventeen years of life and friendship. These items had been carefully and deliberately selected with love, sitting in the tall grass on the side of the highway. They looked out of place. They carried emotional weight and represented the life of a person that shouldn't be gone yet.

I still get a wave of nostalgia when I drive by the crash site today. My chest feels tight. Heavy. I think of Sarah every single time. I always glance into the ditch hoping to spot a cross or memorial marker. The rest of the world drives past that place day after day, like it's just another patch of highway, but for me it's noteworthy. It's where everything changed. For me, that stretch of road is preserved in time, with imaginary scenes of the crash replaying in my mind. It's difficult to describe. It's a peculiar mix of pain and survival, loss and resilience, all linked to a piece of road that most of society overlooks.

On the 100th day after my car crash, I slid into the driver's seat and drove for the first time since June 12th. I had been in a vehicle several times as a passenger, but actually driving hit me differently. It was a big step... a nerve-wracking step. And it was another win for me. It was about autonomy, regaining my independence and proving to myself that I could prevail. Healing wasn't fast or easy, but victories like these reminded me of the progress I had made.

When I ultimately walked into school that fall as a senior, it felt like it was more than just the first day of classes. It felt like reclaiming a piece of my life. I was hopeful that I could still be a normal teenager, and I could finish high school with the class I had grown up with.

However, I didn't feel like the same person I was before the crash, and I wasn't sure how others would see me either. When I was voted homecoming queen by my peers, it wasn't about a crown or a fancy title. It was about acceptance, love and realizing that I was still me. That's when I recognized that people saw me as more than just "that girl who was in that bad car crash." I was more than my scars, my trauma and the struggle I was still fighting. They saw my strength and my perseverance. They saw *me*.

My mom and I went dress and shoe shopping the day I found out I was voted queen. I picked out a long, sparkly, blue, one-shoulder dress. Buying shoes, especially dress shoes after a partial foot amputation, was one of the most difficult things. Being only 17 years old, wanting to wear what I used to wear and do the things everyone else was doing, made it hard. My mom was incredibly supportive, acknowledged the challenge and helped me conquer not only this obstacle but every single one to come.

Within the first several months of being home, I had numerous orthopedic problems with my right knee. I had recurrent bleeding into my knee joint that caused severe pain, swelling and the inability to walk. I felt like I was taking steps backwards, instead of forward.

The first time this happened, I was in the guidance counselor, Mrs. Toney's, office. I recall sitting there talking to her when suddenly my right knee swelled up unprovoked. The size difference between my two knees was extreme and visible through my jeans. I couldn't move it or walk as it was so painful.

The course of the next several months was not easy. My knee tested my patience, my determination and my strength. There were days I felt discouraged, but I kept showing up. Each procedure, each rehab session, each step forward brought with it fortitude and eventually healing.

Following the crash, the extensive scars across my entire abdomen told my story of survival. They were reminders of everything I had been through, but they also carried physical and emotional weight. Weight that I had to learn to accept.

About a year after healing, I had reconstructive surgery to repair those scars. It wasn't about erasing the past or what happened. It was about reclaiming confidence in my new body and learning to see myself with grace and compassion. The scars are forever a part of me. But they now feel less like open wounds and more like a badge of resilience.

I wear my scars proudly. They're not flaws. They're proof I survived. Don't hide your imperfections. They're what make you authentic, relatable and wonderfully human.

Learning to live with a partial foot amputation was also a part of my battle and part of my story. It changed so much. How I moved, how I felt about myself and how I saw the world. But it also showed me how steadfast I could be.

Strength isn't just about walking again, it's choosing to move onward, even when it's arduous. It's understanding how to live in a body that carries both trauma and adaptability. It's defying the odds and still showing up with optimism.

I eventually met with an orthotist who started the process to get me a shoe filler prosthetic for my right foot. The shoe filler was meant to fill the vacant end of my right shoe. The first one I received cost $1,200. It proved not to be very comfortable for me, so I typically ended up putting socks in the ends of my shoes. I still do to this day.

As a 17-year-old, I was mostly interested in getting a life-like prosthesis that looked like a real foot. It was made from silicone, was color-matched with my other foot and looked realistic with toenails that could be painted to match the other foot. And it cost $8,000.00.

I tried to hide my foot when I was out in public. I didn't like attention being drawn to me, and I thought the life-like prosthetic was the answer to my problems.

After a year or two, I eventually received the silicone right foot prosthetic. I painted the toenails to match my left foot. I think it was an important thing for me to have when I was younger, as I was very self-conscious of my lack of toes on one foot.

Now that I've grown, matured and my priorities have changed, having a cosmetic prosthetic is no longer a necessity for me. Practicality, functionality, walking without pain and keeping up with my kids are now of more importance.

I recently came across a company called Neotrek, which specializes in custom footwear for everyone, including partial foot amputees. Their designs gave me something I hadn't felt in years, freedom. My custom socks and sandals fit my unique feet perfectly, serving as a perpetual reminder that even after loss, there are new ways to progress forward with strength and confidence.

Fourteen months after the crash, I moved away from home across the state to Eau Claire. Jess and I were randomly assigned college roommates for our freshman year at University of Wisconsin- EC. One of our first days together, we sat and compared scars like badges of honor. Mine from my crash, hers from scoliosis surgery. Hers stretched across her back, mine ran across my belly. They felt like mirror images of each other. Two completely different challenges etched into skin, but both reminders of what we'd endured. There was something strangely comforting in that moment. Together we learned that scars aren't just signs of pain but proof of healing and of resilience.

Jess shared the following with me, "I remember when she showed me her scars from her car accident. I thought she was so brave, and it was nothing short of a miracle that she was spared in that terrible tragedy - spared to be my roommate."

We still call each other "roommate" to this day.

The crash didn't just alter my mind and body, it changed the course of my life. I saw firsthand the impact that nurses had on a patient's journey. The nurses who cared for me in the hospital, as well as my mom being a nurse, were there for me during some of the most adverse and vulnerable moments of my life. Their examples inspired me to follow suit.

Choosing to pursue a career in nursing became a way of turning my pain into purpose. I know what it feels like to be helpless, to rely on others for everything and to wonder if life would ever be simple again. That perspective is something I apply to my work and the way I care for others.

Sometimes the most important steps are the hardest ones to take. Take them anyway.

Considering the level of unimaginable trauma and pain that I went through: the car crash, losing Sarah, nearly dying but recovering against the odds, the single most pivotal moment in my life was the unexpected passing of my mom on June 5, 2011.

At this point Brian and I lived together in our first home. It was a Sunday morning. It also happened to be my parent's 30th wedding anniversary.

I was getting ready in my bathroom, straightening my hair, while Brian was outside mowing the lawn.

My cellphone rang. It was my dad. I talked to my dad a lot, but it was usually my mom calling on her phone, not my dad's. I answered and he asked if both Brian and I were at home. I told him we were, and he asked me to get Brian. I knew something was wrong at this point.

The call disconnected as I hurried down the stairs to the front door to motion for Brian to come inside. I called my dad back, and he asked us to sit down. I sat down hard on the floor of our office near the front of our house.

He then proceeded to explain that mom had slept in my bedroom that night because she had a headache. He checked on her before he left for church that morning, then found her unresponsive in bed when he returned home. He called 911. I held out hope that he was just going to tell me that mom was in the hospital and not doing well.

Instead, he told me that my mom was dead. My 53-year-old, healthy, beautiful, full of life, favorite person in the world mom was dead. The sudden loss was devastating for me, my brother and my dad. Life had changed, again, in an instant, only a week shy of nine years following my crash. I was 26 years old. Out of all the months in a year, June had suddenly become the most difficult by far.

There is a kind of silence that follows a loss like that: her empty bed, her clothes still hung in the closet, her purse. I didn't want to part with any of her things as that made everything feel so final... almost like losing her all over again.

I can still clearly picture writing her obituary with my dad and brother in the loft of the home they built together. I thought, "This can't be happening. I'm not supposed to be writing an obituary for my mom when I'm only 26 years old. My dad isn't supposed to be a widow at the age of 52. My brother is only 23."

One of my closest friends at the time sent a beautiful floral arrangement for my mom's funeral. It included a small, live tansy plant. I still have this very plant today. I've learned that tansy is frequently added to bridal bouquets as symbolism of enduring and eternal love. This was the perfect and most special addition to a day that will forever be engrained in my memory as the day I said goodbye to my mom.

Like the crash, the death of my mom was a dividing point in my life: life before she died and life after she died. It's how I talk about most things to this day. Events are a time frame in relation to my car crash or my mom's death.

I feel closest to my mom when I'm out in nature. I go to Rock Island year after year to feel her presence. I feel her with me when I see a shelf fungus growing on a tree, a curled piece of birch bark lying on the path or a perfectly round mound of green moss.

Losing two of the most memorable people in the world at such a young age gave me perspective on life. There was no planning for these deaths. No preparing myself. I didn't see it coming. There was no way of knowing that the phone call I had with my mom on Saturday evening, the night she died, was the last time I would ever talk to her.

What's important and what really matters can change in an instant.

Make the phone call. Tell them you love them. Go on the trip.

After being together for the better part of our young lives, Brian and I finally got married on February 3, 2013. We had been through a lot together, and it made sense to make it official. I wanted nothing to do with a traditional wedding since my mom wouldn't be there, so I planned a destination wedding on a cruise ship.

I eventually got my dream job as an emergency room nurse at a local hospital. I loved every second of it. It was my calling. Temporarily. Having kids soon changed my calling.

After our wedding, we were ready to start a family. One of the lingering unknowns was whether I would ever be able to have children. My body had been through so much.

When the long-awaited day finally arrived that I heard my child's heartbeat on the ultrasound machine, it felt like a miracle magnifying another miracle.

It took longer than expected, but we eventually had our first son in March of 2015. Just over two years later, we had our second son in March of 2017. I was thrilled with two healthy children but had always longed for a girl. I told Brian I just didn't think we were done yet. He worried that we'd try for a girl and end up with twin boys. I always told him, "That's fine, we'd have four boys then." We had our third child, a girl who we named after my mom, in September of 2021.

Motherhood was something I once feared might never be feasible. And yet here I am as a mother of three healthy children. Every moment, even the hard ones, is something I will never take for granted because I know just how close I came to never having it at all.

Sometimes the weight of all those losses feels oppressive. But I see my mom's strength in myself now, especially as a parent. I hold my children closer, knowing how fragile life can be, and I carry both Sarah and my mom with me in the way I love them.

My mom died less than four years before my first child was born. My children will never know her voice, her laugh, or the way she held me together through so much. They will only know her through my stories. We talk about Sarah and my mom, look at photos of them in my house and celebrate their birthdays.

Since my car crash and receiving over one hundred units of blood, I've become a lifelong blood donor and advocate for blood donation. What many people don't recognize is that my survival wasn't simply due to the expertise of doctors or the miracles of modern medicine. It was also due to the generosity of countless individuals who had taken the time, days or weeks before, to donate blood. Over one hundred units of blood products. Think about that for a moment; that's not just one or two honorable donors, but an entire community of individuals who gave a piece of themselves so that I could have another chance at life.

Blood donation is something most of us don't ponder until it touches us personally. But I am evidence of its potential. The blood donors are the voiceless heroes of my story. Without those donors, I wouldn't be here today, sharing my story, raising my kids, building a future and inspiring others.

That is why I've made it my calling to be a blood donor and an advocate for blood donation. I started donating blood right around the time my mom passed away. I've done it faithfully since. I enjoy scheduling and coordinating local blood drives and encouraging others to donate blood because one pint can mean the difference between life and death. My goal is to give back what I received and to share my story to inspire others to give back.

Being a trauma survivor has shifted the way I see life today. Blood drives aren't just another community event, they're a necessity. They are opportunities for ordinary people to accomplish extraordinary things.

Shortly after we were home from the hospital, my dad started donating blood for the first time in twenty-six years, long before my blood donation journey started. He has turned into a faithful blood donor since my car crash. I love that he donates as much as he does, since he knows firsthand the impact blood can have on saving someone you love.

If you've ever thought about donating blood, I encourage you to do it. It doesn't take long, and it's important.

When I reflect on Sarah all these years later, there is still a part of me that feels seventeen, forever suspended in that moment of loss. In reality, our lives were just starting when everything changed in an instant. Grief and anguish didn't make sense when I was still so young myself.

Sarah is buried at a cemetery in Marion Wisconsin, under a big silver maple tree near the back corner. For years, when the anniversary of our car crash came about, I'd visit her and bring her a message. I would ask Brian to drill a hole into a softball, so I could write her a letter and tuck it inside the hole. I would leave the ball at her grave site each year, for ten years, before I had kids.

To this day, my husband, kids and I visit her several times a year. My kids call it going to "Sarah's house." They enjoy these cemetery stops to see "Aunt Sarah." I typically take a photo at each visit to document the changes of the season and the size of my kids over the years. They like to help clean her gravestone to keep it looking nice.

Visting Sarah's grave with my children isn't always easy, but I feel it's imperative. My kids didn't lose Sarah, but they lost the chance to get to know her. Part of my job is to tell them about her, get them there and share her memory with them. I want them to know that while her life was short and ended too soon, her impact lives on in the way we honor and remember her.

Visiting her grave is about respecting, teaching and reminding my kids that love doesn't end just because life does.

If you've lost people you love, visit them. Whether that means going to a cemetery or an island in the middle of nowhere. Do it. Talk to them. Remember them.

epilogue

To carry the name Tansy, is to carry a legacy of survival, strength and resilience.

In the end, against all expectations, I lived.

They said I had less than a one percent chance of surviving.

Sarah didn't make it. I carry her memories with me every day. The physical scars are reminders, but so are the emotional and conceptual ones. They are part of who I am and remind me just how tenuous life really is.

I lost parts of my body. I lost the life I knew. But I found a new sense of purpose I didn't know existed. I found fortitude. I found a calling.

I was given over one hundred units of blood to keep me alive, and now I give back every chance I get. I speak. I share. I donate.

These forty-three days remodeled everything; how I mother, how I love, how I show up.

I am not the same person I was before the crash.

Because in the wreckage, I found influence and aspiration I didn't know I had, a purpose I never expected, and a tale I will never stop telling with the hope it will change the life of someone who needs to hear it.

about the author

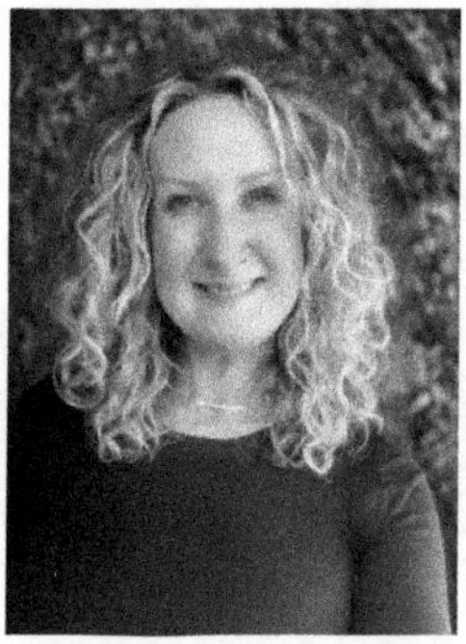

Tansy grew up in the small town of Clintonville, Wisconsin. After surviving a devastating car crash at seventeen that killed her best friend and left her with less than a one percent chance of survival, she went on to find strength, purpose and hope in the years that followed.

Through it all, her middle school sweetheart, Brian stood by her side. The two later married and started a life together.

Inspired by the care she received during her recovery; Tansy pursued a career in nursing and now dedicates her life to helping others and blood donor advocacy.

She and Brian are the proud parents of three healthy children. Her story is a powerful testament to resilience, love and vitality.

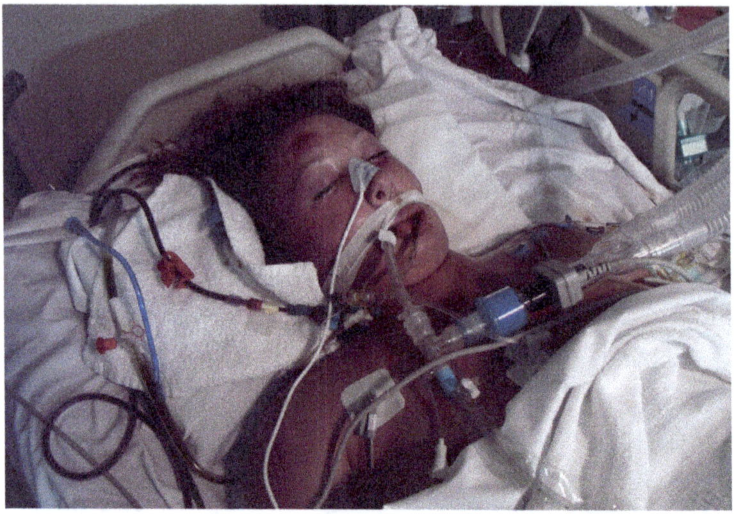

Day 4
This is the first photo taken of my 43-day hospitalization. My body is extremely swollen with extra fluid. Page 21.

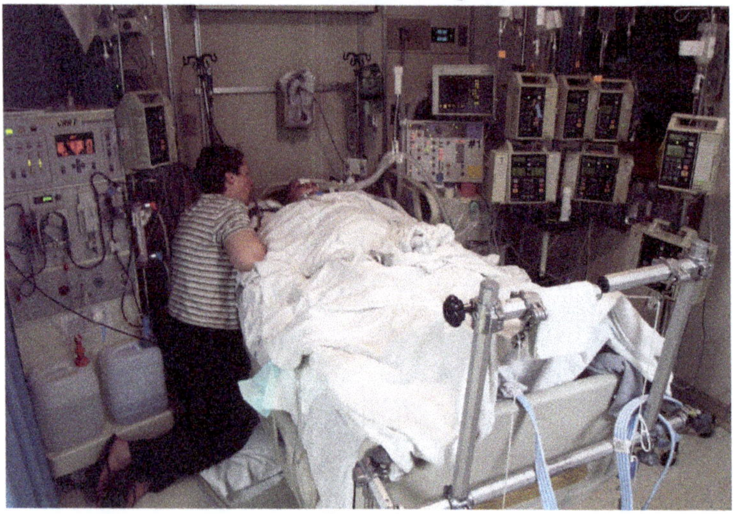

Day 4
My mom, Julie, kneeling at my bedside during one of the most critical and scary moments while my body was failing despite the highest level of life sustaining measures. Page 21-24.

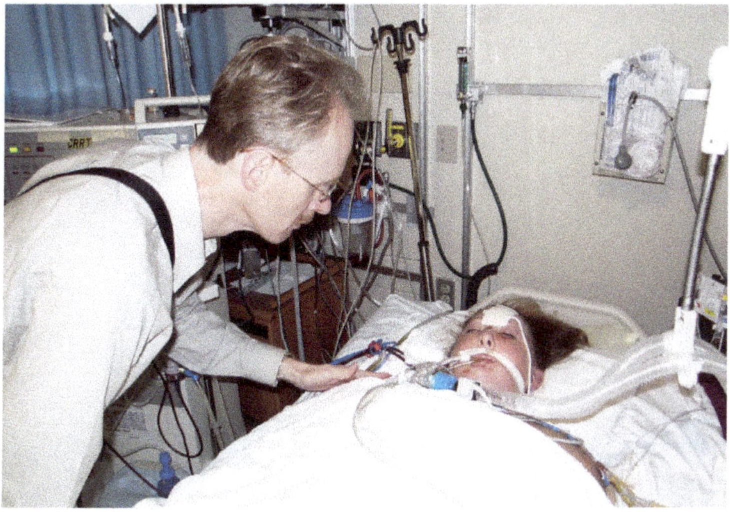

Day 4
My dad, Tim, likely at the request of my mom, pictured with me during what they thought may be their last moments with me. Page 21.

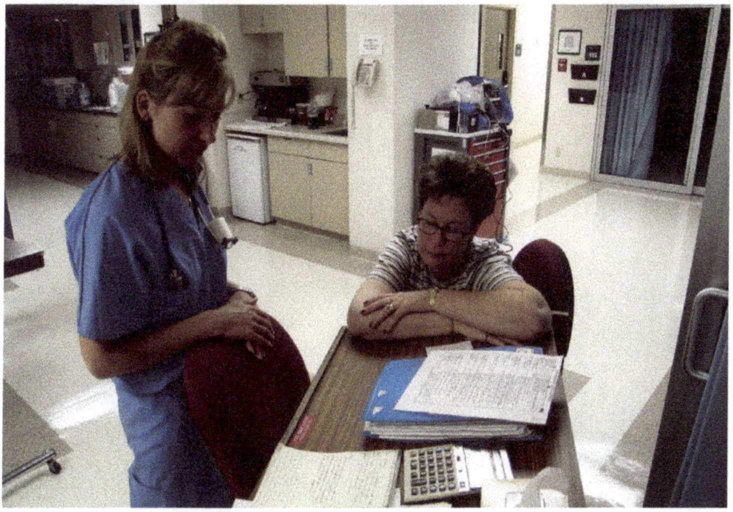

Day 4
My mom and Nurse Sherry, just outside the open door of my critical care room. Page 22.

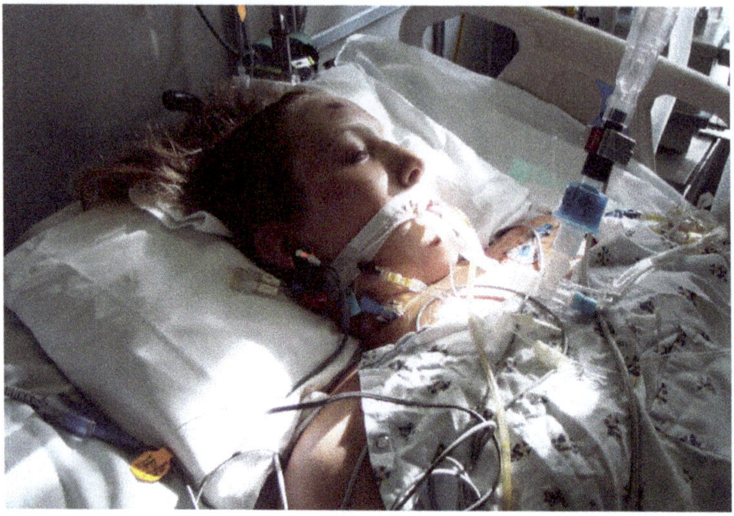

Day 6
June 17, 2002: Still intubated in a medically induced coma but the previously visible swelling has improved significantly. Page 39.

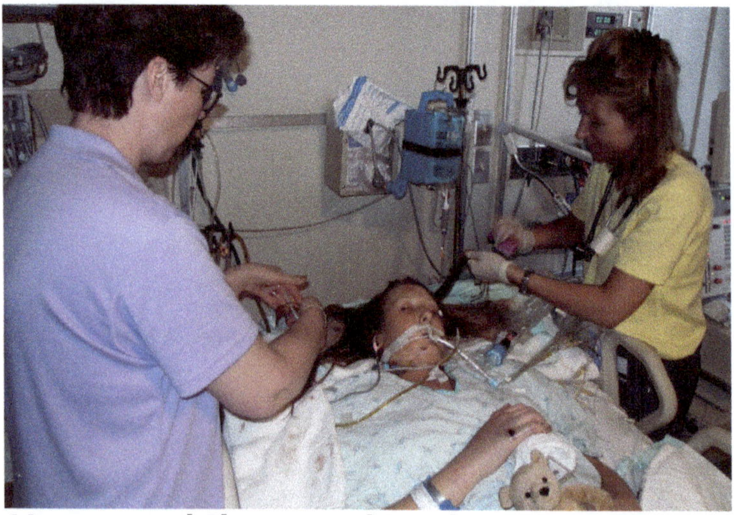

My mom and Sherry combing through my hair for the first time since the crash. Page 30-31.

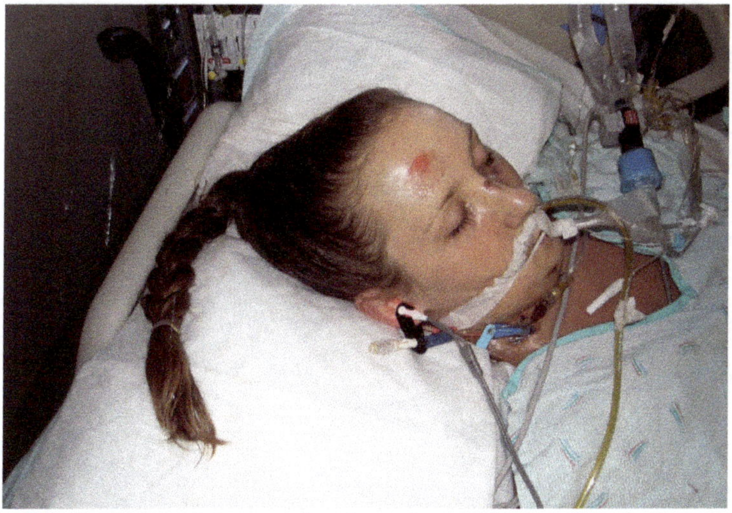

My hair freshly washed and neatly braided. Page 31.

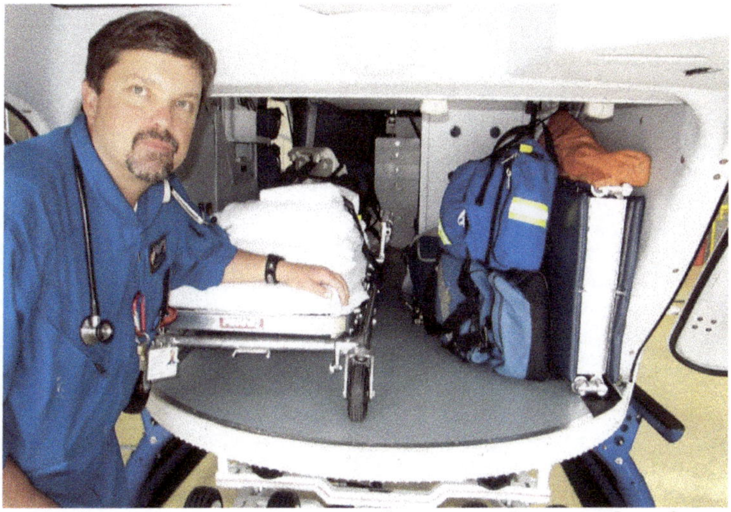

Flight nurse, Jon Hagen showing the inside of Theda Star helicopter.

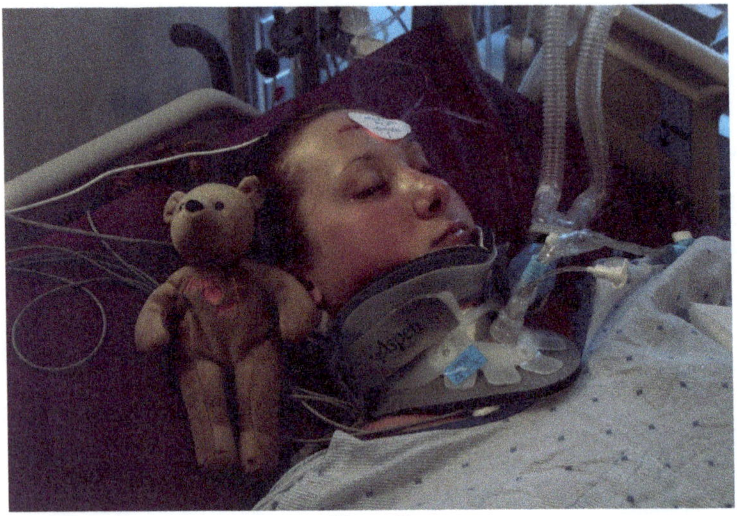

Day 9
I'm no longer intubated as I had a tracheostomy placed a couple days earlier, still in a medically induced coma and on a ventilator. Page 45.

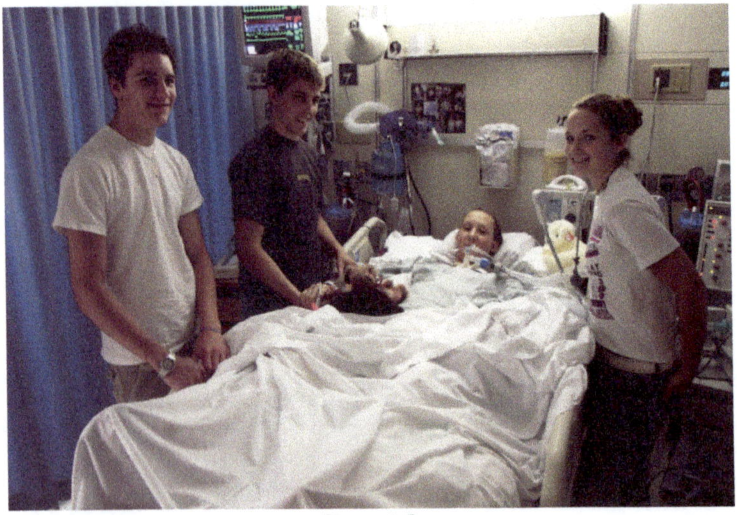

Day 12
Awake with visitors for the first time; my boyfriend Brian and our friends Matt and Becca. Page 60.

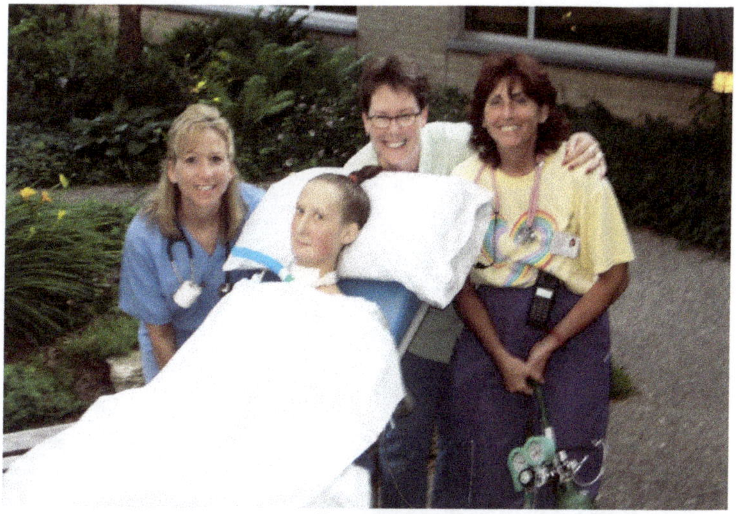

Day 16
Outside in the garden with my nurse Sherry, my mom and respiratory therapist, Sharon. Page 70.

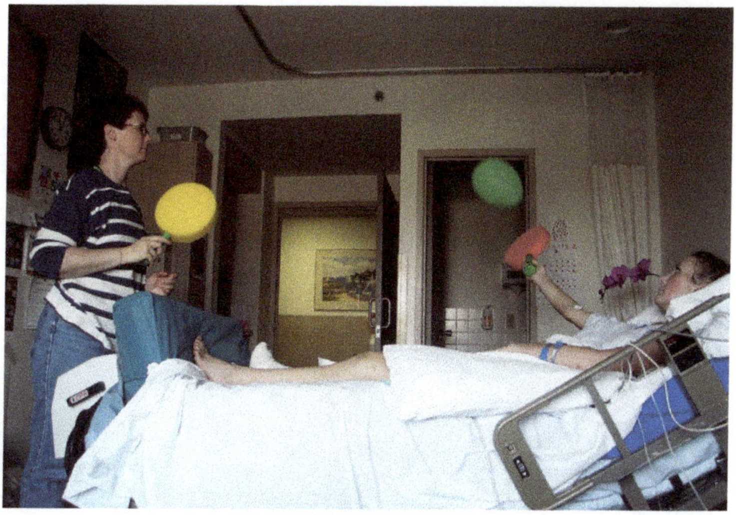

Day 33
Playing balloon ping pong with my mom on the 2nd floor. Page 128.

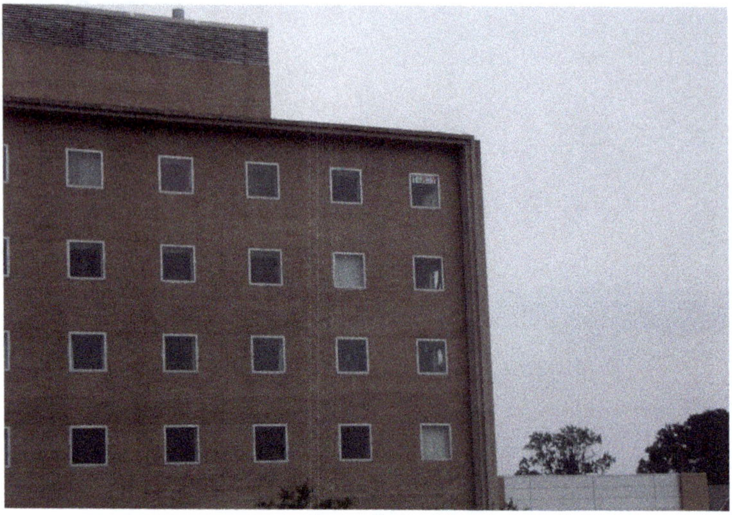

Day 36
A view of my name in the window of my 6th floor rehab room at Theda Clark from the Oak Street Bridge. Page 136.

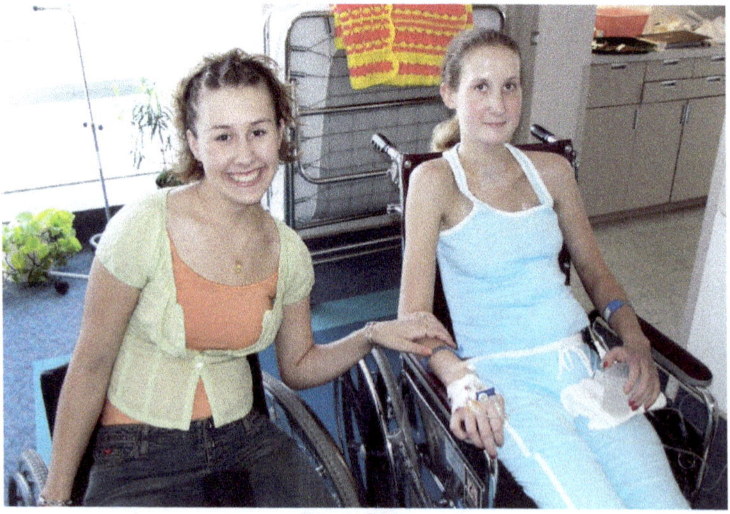

Day 38
The day I met Autumn for the first time. Page 139-140.

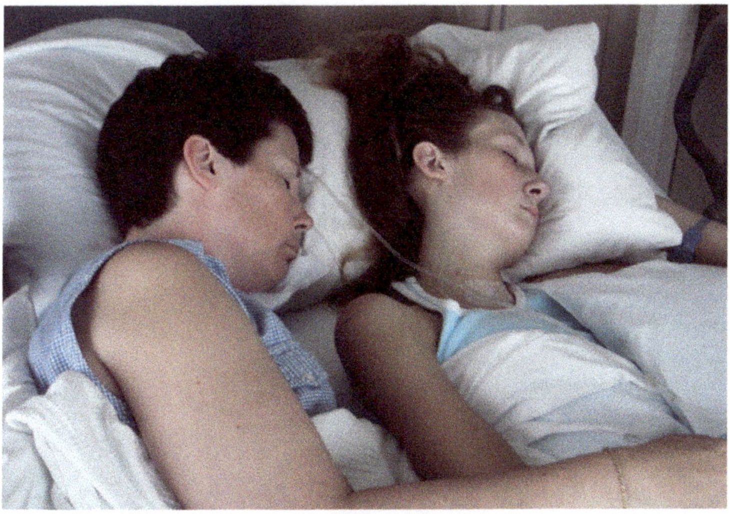

Day 40
My mom and me napping together in my hospital bed on 6th floor. Page 142.

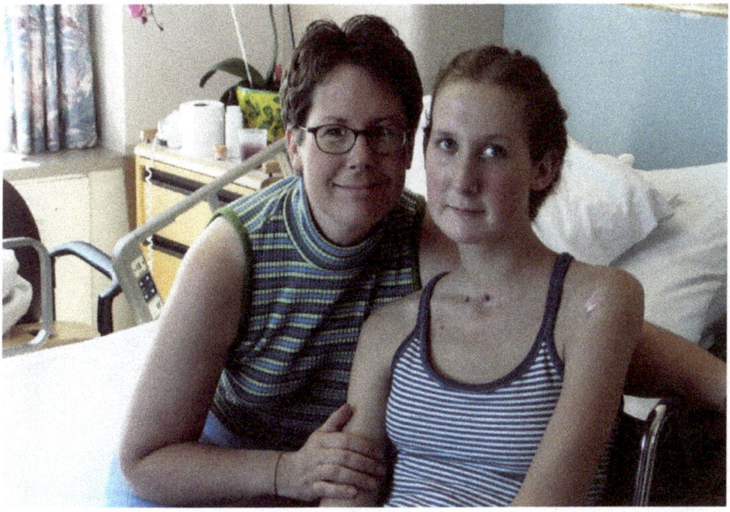

Day 43
July 24, 2002: My mom and me while I'm sitting in a wheelchair ready to be discharged from the hospital. Page 151.

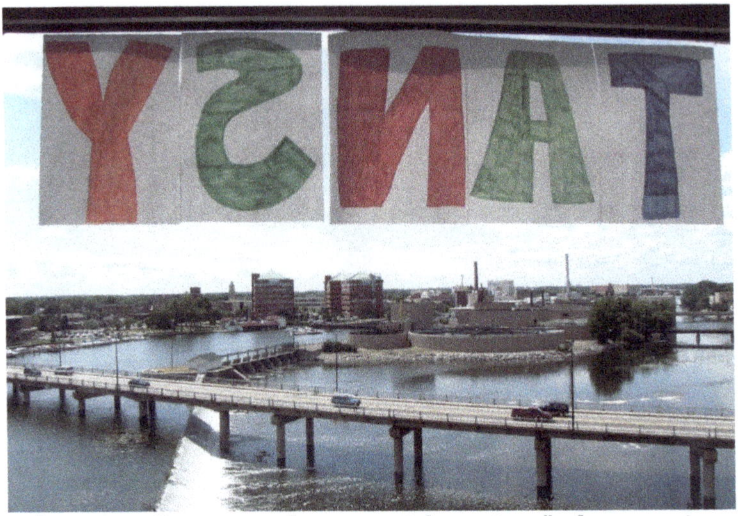

The view from my "room with a view" showcasing my Tansy sign that adorned my window during my stay in rehab.

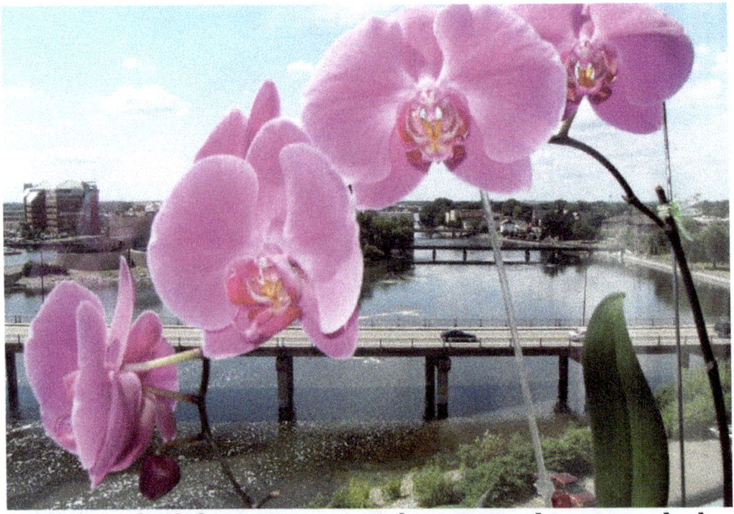

The orchid from my grandparents that traveled with me throughout my hospital stay. Page 85-86.

www.ingramcontent.com/pod-product-compliance
Ingram Content Group UK Ltd.
Pitfield, Milton Keynes, MK11 3LW, UK
UKHW020716041026
15590UKWH00002B/696

9 798994 746608